10[...]
to Boost Your
Immune
System

Theresa Cheung

First published in 2008 by Collins,
an imprint of HarperCollins Publishers Ltd.
77–85 Fulham Palace Road
London
W6 8JB

www.collins.co.uk
Collins is a registered trademark of HarperCollins Publishers Ltd.

8 7 6 5 4 3 2 1
12 11 10 09 08

A catalogue record for this book is available from the British Library.

ISBN 978-0-00-727587-8

Collins uses papers that are natural, renewable and recyclable
products made from wood grown in sustainable forests.
The manufacturing processes conform to the environmental
regulations of the country of origin.

Designed by Martin Brown
Printed and bound in China by Leo Paper

This is a general reference book and although care has been taken
to ensure the information is as up-to-date and accurate as possible,
it is no substitute for professional advice based on your personal
circumstances. Consult your doctor before making any major
changes to your diet. All recipes serve 1 unless otherwise stated.
Both metric and imperial measurements are given for the recipes,
use one set of measures only, not a mixture of both.

CONTENTS

INTRODUCTION

YOUR INVISIBLE ARMY

Without a strong immune system you can't live younger or longer. Your immune system is your invisible army, working tirelessly around the clock to keep you fit and healthy, and fighting off invasion by foreign organisms that can lead to premature ageing and disease.

A vigorous immune system is vital to good health, both physical and mental. Tiredness, frequent colds and other infections, allergies, mood swings and premature ageing are sure-fire signs of a weakened immune system. Learning how to protect and support your immune system is therefore the most important thing you can do for your health and well-being. Fortunately, there are many ways in which you can strengthen and support your immune system – and keep your troops in peak condition – without resorting to the use of antibiotics.

This book gives you all the advice you need to achieve this healthy state of affairs.

So be good to yourself. Read on to discover everything you need to know to stay free from disease and maximise your potential for high-level health, happiness and vitality.

Drawing on a variety of disciplines in medicine and natural health, each immune booster in this book will provide practical strategies you can use in your daily life to strengthen your resistance to illness. And if you do get sick you'll find information that will help you get well faster.

PART ONE:

· ·

UNDERSTANDING YOUR IMMUNE SYSTEM

What is your immune system

· ·

Your immune system is a complex interrelated network of organs, blood cells and chemical reactions that are your body's basic – and mostly highly effective – defence mechanism against invasion from the hordes of bugs (bacteria, viruses, parasites and fungi) that are constantly trying to get inside you.

Every day a healthy body with a fully func-tioning immune system sees off potentially dangerous organisms that can trigger illness, as well as protecting against quirks in your cellular system that might potentially develop into cancerous growths. If your immune defences are working at their optimum level of efficiency, your health is likely to be good. If, however, you feel under par or constantly unwell, this suggests that your immune system is compromised.

Compromised immunity can leave you vulnerable to premature ageing and disease, and impair your ability to heal properly and live your life to the full. It's no surprise that a recent study of healthy centenarians found they had one thing in common: a healthy immune system. A healthy immune system is therefore the key to good health and a long life.

Components of your immune system

The key components of your immune system are the thymus and the lymph system, together with the spleen, bone marrow, white blood cells and antibodies.

The thymus is the source of T cells. T cells – a type of white blood cell or lymphocyte –

are the foot-soldiers of your immune system. They destroy invaders that have been detected by B cells, another type of white blood cell. The lymph system transports nutrients to cells and filters waste. Lymph nodes are collections of lymphoid cells found throughout the body, including the neck, armpits and groin. They are connected by a network of lymph-carrying vessels and are the main sites of storage, activation and production of white blood cells.

The spleen filters the blood, looking out for invaders, and also carries out regular 'MOT checks' on red blood cells. Bone marrow is the source of new red and white blood cells. White blood cells are actually a collection of cells that work together to destroy bacteria and viruses. There are numerous types of white blood cells: leukocytes, helper T cells, natural killer cells and so on. Finally, there are five primary types of antibody, known as 'immunoglobins', each of which responds and binds to a specific invader, preventing it from entering host cells. We need huge quantities of antibodies to protect us from the constant and daily bombardment of bacteria we unknowingly inhale or digest in our food.

How your immune system works

●●

Your immune system is an elaborate, interactive system of cells, chemicals and tissues located throughout your body. When any of its components come into contact with cells or substances – such as bacteria or viruses – to which they are programmed to respond, a series of reactions is triggered that destroys the invaders or renders them harmless.

A cell or chemical that triggers an immune reaction is called an antigen, and that reaction can be either innate or adaptive. The innate immune response produces an immediate, non-specific immune response to disease-causing antigens that enter or appear inside the body. An army of scavenging white blood cells constantly roams around your body on the lookout for bugs; if a white blood cell detects an 'enemy', then it is immediately transported to the nearest lymph node, situated in your neck, armpits and groin, and destroyed without mercy.

You can feel this process happening every time your glands become swollen because innate immunity also includes the inflammation or swelling process.

While the innate response is working on the front lines, the adaptive response system is quietly working behind the scenes to find a defence specifically tailored to deal with the antigen. Typically, the adaptive response takes about five to seven days to get completely mobilised; if the antigen works faster than that, you're in trouble.

Although the immune system is capable of diversifying its defence plan to meet a wide variety of invading antigens – and once immunity to a specific antigen has been developed that immunity will protect against future attacks by antigens that produce similar diseases – it's important to point out that each antigen requires an individual response. So, if you've developed immunity to the chickenpox virus, you still need to develop immunity to deal with the measles virus and if you've developed immunity to one strain of flu virus you still need to develop immunity to deal with countless other cold and flu viruses.

Meet the bugs

Your body is under daily attack from infectious agents doing their best to get inside your body. To a bug, your body offers warmth, safety and food; these make it a very attractive proposition.

Bacteria, viruses and other infectious agents live everywhere. You can find them in the air; on food, plants and animals; in soil and in water; and on almost every surface, including those of your own body. They range in size from microscopic single-cell organisms to parasitic worms that can grow to several centimetres in length.

Most of these agents won't make you ill, but others can cause infection and harm you. Even though your hard-working immune system is powerful and usually successful at defending you from invaders, it does face the constant threat of viruses and bacteria that are forever mutating, and seeking new ways to attack and break down your immune defences. Let's take a look at the constant threats your immune system faces:

Bacteria and viruses

Among the earliest life forms on Earth, bacteria are self-sufficient, one-celled organisms that are visible under a microscope. Not all bacteria, however, are harmful. Some bacteria that live in your body are actually good for you, such as *Lactobacillus acidophilus*, the healthy bacteria that reside in your intestines and help you digest food. But when unhealthy bacteria enter your body they can make you ill by rapidly reproducing and secreting toxic chemicals that can damage cells in the tissue they have invaded. Common conditions caused by bacteria include strep throat and gastrointestinal illness triggered by *E. coli* bacteria, which are often linked to under-cooked meat.

Even smaller than bacteria, viruses can only be seen through electron microscopes, high-powered instruments that are used to study very small objects. Unlike bacteria, viruses are not self-sufficient; they need a suitable host in which to reproduce. When a virus such as influenza enters you it takes over healthy cells and spreads through your body, causing illness.

Fungi and parasites

Slightly larger than bacteria, fungi live in the air, water, soil and on plants. Moulds and yeasts are types of fungi that can live in your body but don't always cause illness. Some fungi such as penicillin – an antibiotic which kills harmful bacteria – have health benefits, but other fungi are not so good for you and can cause illness; an example might be Candida, which can cause yeast infections and oral thrush.

Protozoa are single-celled organisms that spend part of their life cycle outside humans living in food, soil, water or insects, and part of their life cycle living within your body as a parasite. Many protozoa inhabit the intestinal tract and are harmless, but others can cause digestive problems and disease.

Helminths are larger parasites that can enter your body, taking up residence in your intestinal tract where they live off the nutrients in your body. The most common helminths are tapeworms and roundworms.

Signs of infection

Diseases and infections are not the same thing. Infection is the first step to disease when bacteria, viruses or other antigens enter your body and try to multiply and take hold. Disease or illness occur when the cells in your body are damaged by infection, and signs and symptoms of illness will become evident.

Common symptoms of infection, such as sweating, chills, fever, runny nose, sore throat, coughing and sneezing, are all indications that your immune system is doing its job and fighting back. In most cases the natural healing response your immune system offers is effective in warding off invading antigens but sometimes things don't work so efficiently. Bacteria, a virus or other antigens make it past your immune defences and you get ill. And the most common way to get ill is with a cold or flu virus.

The common cold

It's called the common cold for a reason; you are more likely to get a cold than any other type of illness. More than 200 different viruses can cause the common cold and there are very few people who escape the infection each year. Most adults get between two and four colds a year and most children get between three and seven as their immune systems are less well developed.

Colds can occur year round but are most common in winter. Symptoms generally include a runny nose, nasal congestion and sneezing, but you may also have a sore throat, cough, headache and mild fever. When someone is down with a cold, his or her nose is teeming with cold viruses and sneezing, nose blowing and nose wiping all spread the virus. You can catch a cold by sitting close to someone with a cold and inhaling the virus or by touching your eyes, nose and mouth after you have touched something contaminated with the virus. People are typically most contagious for the first three days of the cold and not contagious at all after a week.

Once you have caught a cold, symptoms appear within a few days and typically begin with a scratchy throat, followed by sneezing and watery nasal secretions that gradually turn thicker, becoming yellow and green. Most colds are over in a week, with perhaps a few symptoms – such as a cough – lingering on for a further week.

If you get a cold you don't need antibiotics to treat it unless you have yellow or green nasal discharge for more than 10–14 days. Over-the-counter remedies can offer relief but they won't cure it. It's important to rest and drink plenty of fluids.

Flu

Caused by the influenza virus which gives it its name, the 'flu' which typically arrives in the winter months is a contagious infection of the nose, throat and lungs. It often begins with a fever, raising your body temperature to 39–41°C (about 102–106 °F), and other common symptoms such as body aches, dizziness, lack of energy and a flushed face. The fever can last for up to five days but normally subsides after a day or two.

Sometime around day four of the illness the 'whole body' symptoms subside and respiratory symptoms, such as coughs, sore throats, runny or blocked noses and sneezing, take centre stage. These symptoms tend to continue for about a week, but coughs and tiredness can linger for weeks after the rest of the illness is over.

The influenza virus is airborne and can be caught by breathing in droplets from coughs or sneezes. Most often, however, it is caught when you touch a tap, phone or door handle with the infection on it, and then touch your mouth, nose and eyes.

Millions of people get influenza every year; most recover but for some the symptoms are so severe that they need to be hospitalised. All ages are at risk of serious complications with flu, but those most at risk include babies, children, pregnant women, people over the age of 60, and anyone with diabetes or a chronic heart, lung or kidney condition.

In most people who are otherwise healthy, influenza subsides within seven to ten days. If you do get flu and are not in a high-risk category, resting, using over-the-counter medications that relieve symptoms, drinking plenty of water and avoiding alcohol, tobacco

and antibiotics are the best ways to treat it.
(For more advice on DIY methods to ease
symptoms of colds and influenza, *see* 'Part
Three: Fighting Infection'.)

Is it a cold or flu?

Most people get a cold several times a year but
fortunately, influenza strikes only once every few
years. The flu virus is often mistaken for a cold
virus since both these infections share similar
symptoms, but the two diseases are very different.
For one thing colds tend to go away without
causing trouble but influenza can lead to
complications such as pneumonia. Being able
to spot a case of flu quickly also opens up the
possibility of taking antiviral medications, such
as Tamiflu and Relenza, which can kill the virus
and speed recovery. Once flu is diagnosed, your
doctor can determine which one is best for you.

If you aren't sure if you have a cold or a case
of the flu, bear in mind that colds tend to come on
gradually. The first sign is often a sore or scratchy
throat, followed by a runny nose and sneezing.

Other symptoms include coughing, headaches and stuffiness. Also colds don't usually cause fevers in adults, although they can sometimes do so in children. The flu, on the other hand, leads quickly to a high fever and the symptoms tend to be far more severe. You might feel weak, tired and drained of all energy, and you might also experience chills, a sore throat, strong headaches and aches and pains (including eye pains).

A word about bird flu

Known as 'avian influenza', bird flu is a viral disease caused by different strains of the influenza virus. It mostly infects birds. Recent outbreaks in Europe have largely been caused by a highly contagious and virulent strain of the virus known as 'H5N1'. At present, H5N1 is only mildly infectious to humans who have been in contact with infected birds and it cannot be transmitted from one human to another. However, virus experts fear that the H5N1 virus could mutate and be transferred to humans, or combine with other influenza viruses already infecting humans, causing a 21st-century flu pandemic on the scale of the 'Spanish flu' that followed World War I, which killed over 50 million people worldwide.

Research suggests that flu drugs, such as Relenza and Tamiflu, are effective treatments for the disease, although there is concern that such drugs may not be as readily available or as effective as hoped if the virus mutates. In addition, a number of companies are trying to develop a vaccine, although this is proving difficult as the flu virus mutates frequently and the vaccines need to be constantly modified.

Despite growing concern, health experts strongly advise the public not to panic as there is no immediate threat to humans. The World Health Organisation (WHO) has effective disease-control measures in place in areas where outbreaks have occurred or are likely to occur. Currently, the WHO is also creating an emergency plan to handle a pandemic and governments are stockpiling antiviral medications. The best way to protect yourself is to keep your immune system as strong as possible by following the guidelines in this book and by staying away from infected birds.

Auto-immune disorders

A weakened immune system will not only increase your susceptibility to colds and flu, it can also increase your risk of auto-immune disorders in which the immune system attacks healthy body cells.

Normally the immune system is capable of telling the difference between 'self' and 'non-self' tissue, but auto-immune disorders occur when it can no longer differentiate between the two. Why this happens is still uncertain. Some experts believe that these disorders occur following infection by some kind of organism that looks similar to particular cells in the body, which are later mistaken for the organism and targeted for attack.

In many cases, auto-immune disorders cause the destruction of body tissue, resulting in the decreased functioning of an organ or tissue, or several organs or tissues. Examples of auto-immune disorders include:

Chronic fatigue syndrome: A condition of prolonged weariness and fatigue that is not relieved by rest or caused by other medical conditions. Experts aren't sure what causes it but one theory is that it is caused by some sort of auto-immune response.

Diabetes (Type 1): A disease that occurs when the pancreas produces too little insulin to regulate blood sugar. Symptoms include increased thirst, weight loss, fatigue and increased urination.

Multiple sclerosis: An auto-immune disease that affects the central nervous system (brain and spinal cord). Symptoms include fatigue, tremors and weakness in one or more extremities.

Pernicious anaemia: Caused by the lack of a substance needed to absorb vitamin B12 from the gastrointestinal track. Symptoms include fatigue, unsteady gait and bleeding gums.

Rheumatoid arthritis: A painful long-term disease that causes inflammation of the joints and surrounding tissues.

Most auto-immune disorders are chronic but can be controlled with medication. The outcome of treatment will vary with the disorder but the aim is to reduce the immune response against normal body tissue while leaving intact the immune response against invading antigens.

Allergies

Allergic disorders occur when the immune system over-reacts to exposure to substances in the environment and triggers defence mechanisms such as swelling, watery eyes and sneezing. The substances that provoke this over-reaction are called allergens, and over-reactions to allergens are typically controlled by medications called antihistamines.

When an allergen enters the body of a person with a sensitive immune system, histamine and other chemicals are released by certain cells. It is these that cause itching, swelling, watery mucus production, skin rashes and other symptoms. Such symptoms are inconvenient and unpleasant but are not life-threatening; treatment generally involves the use of medications, such as antihistamines. Sufferers can also take steps to reduce their exposure to known allergens.

The most common allergic disorders include:

Asthma: A respiratory disorder that involves an allergic response by the lungs and can cause breathing problems. If the lungs are sensitive to certain allergens, such as pollen or dust mites, this can trigger a narrowing of the breathing tubes in the lungs, making it hard for the person to breathe. Asthma symptoms can also be triggered by respiratory infections, exercise, cold air, stress, smoke and other pollutants.

Eczema: An over-sensitive reaction that occurs in the skin and causes a scaly, itchy rash. Exposure to environmental irritants can worsen symptoms, as can dry skin, exposure to water, temperature changes and stress. Consult your doctor for a diagnosis of eczema because it can be hard to differentiate from other skin disorders.

Food allergies (to products such as nuts), **seasonal allergies** (such as hay fever) and **environmental allergies** (to organisms such as dust mites). All of these are also caused by an over-sensitive immune system, which leads to an incorrect immune response when the immune system reacts to allergens or substances that are generally harmless.

Improving your immunity

A large number of health problems can be linked to an under-par immune system. On the surface, the symptoms of hay fever may seem quite different from the painful, inflamed joints of arthritis or the wheezing of asthma. They are all triggered, however, by an immune system that is struggling to cope with the pressures being placed on it.

There are a number of reasons why your immune system may be compromised or struggling. It is important to understand that in the majority of cases your immunity can be weakened or strengthened by factors within your control. Although the immune system is less efficient in children and the elderly, even the most susceptible person can boost their immune system by:

- keeping up to date with vaccinations
- avoiding common enemies of immunity
- heeding the warning signs of an immune system under pressure
- making the right diet and lifestyle choices.

Vaccination

Your doctor can help you stay healthy by offering you appropriate vaccinations to reduce your risk of getting infected with diseases that are potentially life-threatening. Many vaccines are given in childhood, but adults can also be vaccinated to prevent illness such as tetanus and influenza.

Your body can become immune to bacteria, viruses and other germs by getting a disease – this is called natural immunity. Immunity can also be developed through vaccines – vaccine-induced immunity. Vaccines work by stimulating an immune response without causing disease. Several doses of a vaccine may be needed for a full immune response and it should be noted that vaccines are not free of possible side effects, which often include swelling at the injection site or a mild fever.

Vaccines are the first line of defence against diseases such as polio, measles, tetanus, mumps, rubella, influenza and diphtheria. Were it not for the widespread use of vaccines, a far greater number of deaths would have occurred in childhood, and a great many more people would be living with the chronic and crippling after-effects of disease.

Despite the proven benefits of vaccines there is public concern about their safety and possible side effects, but vaccination continues to be strongly recommended by doctors because gaining natural immunity involves considerable risk.

Vaccination is generally considered by health experts to be the right thing to do as it protects you as well as others. If you have any concerns about vaccinations for which you or your child are eligible, however, it is important to discuss them with your doctor before you come to an informed decision. You can also look at the following website: **www.immunisation.nhs.uk**. This is an up-to-date source of information on vaccines, disease and immunisation in the UK. Whatever you decide, remember that the overwhelming majority of evidence and research suggests that vaccinations save lives.

The flu jab

Catching flu is tough for most people but for some, especially the elderly, it can lead to serious illnesses such as bronchitis and pneumonia that may lead to hospital treatment and – in severe cases – death. That's why doctors advise all people over the age of 65, and those with long-term medical conditions, to have a yearly flu vaccination.

The best time to have a flu jab is between late September and early November, to prepare for the winter months. The flu virus mutates frequently, which is why yearly jabs are advised to guarantee protection against the latest strain of the virus. If you think you need a flu vaccination, check with your doctor or ask your local pharmacist for advice. Bear in mind that it takes between seven and ten days for the vaccine to take effect, and that the flu jab doesn't stop you catching the many other viruses that appear every winter.

Immunity enemies

Although compromised immunity can be triggered by accidents and medication (or in rare cases, immuno-deficiency disease viruses such as HIV), the most common causes of below-par immunity are in fact related to diet and lifestyle choices. In other words, the strength of your immune system is strongly influenced by factors within your control.

A healthy immune system forms the basis of your well-being, so making it more efficient by avoiding anything that might compromise or weaken it is fundamental to good health. Listed below are factors that clinical experience and modern research have shown to have the most damaging influence on immunity, and which should be avoided to ensure good health.

Nutritional deficiencies: The immune system works best when you keep it supplied with a full range of micronutrients such as vitamins and minerals. A poor diet increases the likelihood of nutritional deficiencies and therefore weakens immunity. (For advice on optimising your immunity through diet choices, see 'Part Two: Boosting immunity with nutrition'.)

Stress: Chronic stress causes the adrenal glands to secrete higher levels of corticosteroids, which depress immune function. (For advice on boosting your immunity through stress management, see 'Part Two: Boosting immunity with lifestyle changes'.)

Depression: Research shows that people who are negative, moody, nervous and easily stressed have a weaker immune response than those who are more positive. (For advice on boosting your immunity with a positive attitude, see 'Part Two: Boosting immunity with a Fighting spirit'.)

Lack of quality sleep: Lack of sleep seems to impair the healthy functioning of the immune system. (For advice on getting a good night's sleep, see 'Part Two, pages 92–93'.)

Sedentary lifestyle: Exercise enhances the overall functioning of the immune system, and protects against heart disease, cancer and osteoporosis, as well as being an effective way to relieve stress. Research has shown that people who exercise regularly are less likely to get colds than those who are not active. (For advice on immune boosting and exercise, see 'Part Two, pages 94–95'.)

Over-exertion: Too much exercise can be as damaging as too little. Over-exertion suppresses T-cell function and other immune responses. (For advice on boosting immunity with a regular, moderate exercise plan, *see* 'Part Two, pages 94–101'.)

Weight gain: Obesity increases the risk of cancer and heart disease, so maintaining a healthy body weight is a sensible way to encourage long-term immune health, as well as general well-being. (For advice on boosting immunity through weight management, *see* 'Part Two, pages 102–103'.)

Alcohol, cigarettes and drugs: Alcohol in excess, together with smoking and taking recreational drugs are simply not compatible with a healthy immune system. The odd drink now and again is fine, but more than one drink a day depresses the immune system; drug use is a major cause of poor nutrition, which damages immunity further; and cigarette smoke contains high levels of dangerous chemicals, including cadmium, which is a powerful immune system depressant. (For advice on quitting smoking, *see* 'Part Two, page 126'.)

Over-use of antibiotics: Over-use of antibiotics can cause unintentional suppression of normal immune system responses. (For advice on the sensible use of antibiotics, *see* 'Part Three: Fighting Infection'.)

Environmental pollutants: All of the following three categories can compromise immunity and although it is impossible to avoid them completely, sensible use and taking the recommended precautions are advised.

- Radiation: From mobile phones, televisions, microwaves, radio transmitters and computers.
- Chemicals: From engine exhaust fumes, pesticides, herbicides, smoke, aerosols, paints and household products such as air fresheners, cosmetics, deodorants, detergents and furniture polish. Food additives, preservatives and colourings also fall into this category.
- Biological: From house dust, dust mites and mould.

(For advice on avoiding environmental pollutants that can compromise immunity, *see* 'Part Two, pages 146-167'.)

Is your immune system in trouble?

••

The earlier you recognise the signs and symptoms of weakened immunity, the faster you can take corrective action and decrease your risk of illness or poor health. Your immune system may be invisible but there are ways to tell if it is in trouble. Use the checklist below to see if your immune system is in need of a boost.

❏ Do you feel as if you have lost your energy or get-up-and-go?
❏ Do you feel the cold more than other people?
❏ Do you get more than two or three colds a year?
❏ Have you noticed a loss of libido?
❏ Are you overweight?
❏ Do you smoke?
❏ Is your job sedentary?
❏ Do you spend little time in natural sunlight?
❏ Is your diet high in sugar and refined processed foods?

- Do you feel stressed, up and down or just below par?
- Are you forgetful?
- Is it ages since you had a good night's sleep?
- Do you need coffee or other stimulants to get you through the day?
- Is your skin dry or dull?
- Do you suffer from indigestion, constipation or bouts of diarrhoea?
- Is your neck stiff and sore when you move?
- Does your breath smell?
- Do you suffer from bleeding gums?
- Do you suffer from eye strain?
- Do you suffer from frequent headaches?
- Can you sometimes hear high-pitched sounds in your ears?
- Do you suffer from allergies?
- Do you get food cravings or feelings of intense hunger?
- Are you prone to thrush or cystitis?
- Do your cuts or wounds heal slowly?
- Do you suffer from anaemia?
- Does your hair lack shine?
- Do you often feel fed-up and run down?

If you ticked more than 5 boxes and you can't find any logical explanation (for example, a stiff neck is to be expected if you slept in a draught; hunger is normal if you haven't eaten for a few hours and so on), your immune system is definitely in need of a boost. Follow as much of the advice as you can in 'Part Two: 100 Immune System Boosters'.

If you answered 'yes' to only a few questions, your immune system is doing its job well, but it's still worthwhile reviewing 'Part Two' to find ways to turn any 'yes' answers you gave into 'no' answers.

Making immune-boosting diet and lifestyle choices

Danger comes when your immune system is weakened, and invaders remain undetected and start to multiply. Some invaders are so powerful that they trample your body's immune system, but in the great majority of cases research has shown that making the right diet and lifestyle choices is the most effective way to boost your immunity and protect your health.

Although vaccinations are a good insurance policy against disease, and medications can save lives, the first line of defence against unpleasant illnesses – such as colds and influenza – is to make sure your immune system is as strong and healthy as possible. The 100 immune-system boosters that follow will give you all the information you need to keep your body's defences strong through informed diet and lifestyle choices. And whether you decide to incorporate one or all 100 boosters into your life, bear in mind that each one is designed not only to keep you as free from illness as possible, but to also help you feel great, look better and live longer.

PART TWO:

100 IMMUNE SYSTEM BOOSTERS

Boosting immunity with nutrition

1 Go Mediterranean

If you keep your body well nourished with a healthy, balanced diet, you can literally 'eat yourself well'.

Nutrients are needed for every part of your immune system, and for renewal, repair and defence against infection and illness, so its strength will depend on the quality of your diet.

It is therefore important to maintain a healthy, balanced diet that provides an adequate intake of vitamins, minerals and dietary fibre.

But what is a healthy, balanced diet? Studies have shown that the so-called 'Mediterranean diet' can offer protection against obesity, heart disease, osteoporosis, cancer and diabetes.

The Mediterranean diet is rich in fruits, vegetables and wholegrains, and contains adequate amounts of oily fish, nuts, seeds, legumes, diary products, lean meat or meat substitutes. Saturated fat, salt and sugar intake are limited, and processed, refined foods are off the menu entirely. Olive oil, the primary source of fat in the Mediterranean diet, is an excellent source of monounsaturated fatty acids that help to lower cholesterol. It is also rich in vitamins and antioxidants that fight cancer and lower the risk of developing degenerative diseases.

In a nutshell, research suggests that the Mediterranean diet, with its emphasis on a wide variety of fresh whole foods – along with the odd glass of antioxidant-rich red wine – is the template for a healthy immune-boosting diet.

2 Double take

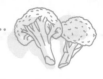

The nutritional benefit that you receive from fruits and vegetables is unparalleled.

Experts advise eating five to nine servings of fruits and vegetables per day; one way to maximise the variety of immune-boosting vitamins, minerals, fibre and antioxidants, is to make sure you eat two different colours of vegetables and fruits with each meal.

Each different-coloured fruit and vegetable contains unique health components that are essential to our health. The phrase 'eating a rainbow of fruits and vegetables' is a simple way of remembering to get as much colour variety in your diet as possible, so that you can maximise your intake of a broad range of nutrients.

Red: Tomatoes, berries, peppers and radishes contain nutrients that can reduce the risk of prostate cancer, lower blood pressure, reduce tumour growth and cholesterol levels, eliminate harmful free radicals, and support joint tissue in arthritis cases.

Orange and yellow: Carrots, yams, squash, oranges, papayas and other orange and yellow fruits and vegetables contain nutrients that can reduce age-related macular degeneration and the risk of prostate cancer, lower cholesterol and blood pressure, promote collagen formation and healthy joints, fight harmful free radicals and work with magnesium and calcium to build healthy bones.

White: Mushrooms, pak choi and pumpkins contain nutrients that can activate natural killer B and T cells, reduce the risk of colon, breast and prostate cancers, and balance hormone levels, reducing the risk of hormone-related cancers.

Green: Kale, spinach, cabbage, alfalfa sprouts, mustard greens and collard greens are all examples of green vegetables that contain nutrients that can reduce cancer risk, lower blood pressure and cholesterol levels, boost digestion, support retinal health and vision, fight harmful free radicals, and boost immune system activity.

Blue and purple: Blueberries, pomegranates, grapes, elderberries, aubergines and prunes contain nutrients that boost healthy digestion and act as anti-carcinogens in the digestive tract.

3 Drink your lemons

Drinking a glass of lemon juice diluted with filtered water every morning is the perfect way to kick-start your digestion and boost your immunity at the same time.

Lemons contain bioflavonoids, a group of nutrients that boosts immunity by protecting the cells of your body against environmental pollutants. Along the membrane of each cell there are microscopic parking spaces, called receptor sites. Pollutants, toxins or germs can park here and gradually eat their way into the membrane of the cell, but when bioflavonoids fill up these parking spots there is no room for toxins to park. Bioflavonoids also reduce cholesterol's ability to form plaques in arteries and lessen the formation of microscopic arterial blood clots, which can lead to heart attacks and strokes. Studies have shown that people who eat the most bioflavonoids have less cardiovascular disease.

Lemon is also the ideal food for restoring the acid-alkali balance in your body. Drinking freshly squeezed lemon juice in water first thing in the morning or adding it to tea, salad dressings (in place of vinegar), baking or cooking, helps maintain your body's internal balance at a pH that supports healthy bacteria, instead of the viruses and harmful bacteria that thrive in more acidic environments. Apple cider vinegar is another great way to improve your body's alkalinity, but the taste of lemons is much more pleasant!

Fresh lemon juice drink

To make a glass of fresh lemon juice, squeeze the juice of one lemon into a glass, add 300 ml (10 fl oz) pure, filtered, slightly warm water and 1 teaspoon of maple syrup for sweetness. Stir and drink immediately. Remember, first thing in the morning about fifteen minutes before breakfast is the optimum time to drink lemon juice.

4 Alkalise, alkalise, alkalise

Your immune system is strongest in an alkaline environment. Many bacteria and viruses love an acid environment, but cannot survive in a healthy alkaline state. If you're feeling run down, eating lots of green vegetables and drinking plenty of water will boost alkalinity and therefore your immunity.

Your immune system relies on water. It carries nutrients to the cells, carries waste, bacteria and toxins away from the cells and out of the body, keeps body temperature stable, protects joints and keeps the lining of your mouth hydrated and moist, reducing susceptibility to colds.

Don't wait until you're thirsty to drink water, as thirst is – along with headaches and dark yellow urine (healthy urine is pale yellow) – a sign of dehydration. Your body's need for water is constant and experts recommend that you drink six to eight glasses a day, more if you are sweating, exercising or if the weather is hot. And it's best to drink filtered water only, as tap water may be contaminated by lead and other toxins that your body doesn't want or need.

5 A yoghurt a day

Look for yoghurt that contains live active cultures indicating helpful bacteria and try to eat one every day for breakfast or dessert, or use live yoghurt in salad dressings, smoothies and dips.

A live natural yoghurt per day might help keep infections at bay. That's because these yoghurts contain probiotics – bacteria that stimulate immunity cells in the gastrointestinal tract (GI). Normal, healthy bacteria that colonise the GI tract help you resist bad bacteria and detoxify harmful substances. In addition to their protective effect in the GI tract, probiotics may also help stimulate immune-cell production system-wide. In a recent study of 33 women from the University of Vienna, those who ate yoghurt daily for two weeks raised their immune-boosting T-lymphocyte cell count by nearly 30 per cent. (*See* 'Part Three, pages 217–19 for advice on taking probiotic supplements.)

6 FOS power

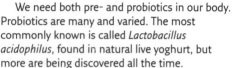

A bowl of oatmeal porridge or shredded wheat for breakfast will give your immune system a much-needed prebiotic fix.

We need both pre- and probiotics in our body. Probiotics are many and varied. The most commonly known is called *Lactobacillus acidophilus*, found in natural live yoghurt, but more are being discovered all the time.

Prebiotics – also known as FOS (Fructo-oligo-saccharides) – on the other hand, are a kind of natural fibre that nourishes and supports the good work of friendly bacteria, or probiotics. Prebiotics occur naturally in foods such as garlic, onions, leeks, shallots, asparagus, spinach, Jerusalem artichokes, chicory, peas, beans, lentils, oats and bananas. Including more of these foods in your diet will therefore be giving both your digestive system and your immunity a boost. One of the best ways to ensure you are getting enough FOS power in your diet is to have oatmeal, shredded wheat or another wholegrain cereal for breakfast.

7 Good coffee habits

Coffee doesn't help your
immune system do its job
efficiently, so keep your coffee
consumption down to no more than
two cups a day.

The caffeine in coffee can temporarily boost
alertness, perk up performance and possibly
even improve concentration. But before you
pour yourself another cup, experts say it's
important to remember coffee's main ingredient,
caffeine, is a drug and not a nutrient necessary
for good health, such as vitamins and minerals.
Caffeine can also dehydrate you and leach
important immune-boosting nutrients, such as
bone-boosting calcium, out of your body. In fact,
too much caffeine may also lead to health
problems, such as high blood pressure, brittle
bones, sleep disorders and just plain irritability.

You don't have to stop drinking coffee
altogether, but, if you are drinking more than
three cups of coffee a day, you do need to cut it
down to one or two cups. Here are some tips to
make sure your coffee-drinking habits are healthy:

- When you drink your coffee, make sure you add an additional glass of water to your daily water intake per cup of coffee to avoid its dehydrating effects.
- Drinking one to three cups of coffee a day (up to 300 mg of caffeine) does not seem to have any negative effects in most healthy people. However, pregnant women, children, people with heart disease or peptic ulcers and the elderly may be more susceptible to the effects of caffeine, and are therefore advised to restrict their intake.
- Be aware that the caffeine content of coffee varies widely depending on roasting and brewing methods, as well as the size of the cup from which you're drinking. For example, a recent study showed that a 475 ml (16 fl oz) cup of the house blend at a leading coffee chain had a massive average of 259 mg of caffeine.
- Put back some of those lost nutrients by adding two tablespoons of milk to your coffee or making your espresso a latte.

Coffee is the main source of caffeine for many people, but other items, such as soft drinks, tea, chocolate, and cold and headache medicines also contain caffeine and can add substantially to your daily caffeine quota. As for chocolate (another source of caffeine), make sure that the type you eat is quality dark chocolate, containing at least 70 per cent cocoa solids.

Some people feel the buzz of caffeine more than others. Listen to your body and know when to say 'no' to that extra cup of coffee, even if you are surrounded by people who drink it like water.

It is important to bear in mind that coffee drinkers who skip their daily fix may experience temporary caffeine withdrawal (usually in the form of a headache or drowsiness), but that these symptoms will disappear within 24–48 hours.

8 Sugar shut down

The next time you're tempted to grab a bar of chocolate, down a sugary drink or tuck into a sugary cereal, give your immune system a break and have a piece of fruit or a bowl of oatmeal instead.

The impact of refined white sugar on your immune system can be enormous. Eating or drinking 100 grams (8 tablespoons) of sugar – the equivalent of about two cans of a full-sugar fizzy drink – can reduce the ability of your white blood cells to kill germs by 40 per cent. The immune-suppressing effect of sugar starts less than 30 minutes after ingestion and may last for up to 5 hours. On top of all this, a diet high in sugar increases your risk of blood-sugar imbalances that can trigger mood swings, weight gain, fatigue, headaches, hormonal imbalances and a host of other unpleasant symptoms.

If you do only one thing to boost your immune system, eliminating sugar will do the trick. Sugar gives you no nutrients, just calories. You will see noticeable results in your energy levels, weight distribution, immunity and ability to think clearly when you break the cravings and stop eating refined sugar.

Cutting down on your sugar intake may seem daunting at first, but it is easier than you think if you follow these tips to total sugar shut-down:

Sweet substitutes: Try fruits and unsweetened fruit juices more often in meals and snacks to cut down on sugar. Fruits have natural sugars, but they also give you important vitamins and minerals. Plan to have fresh fruit in season for desserts. Use dried fruits to sweeten cereals and baked goods. Slice a banana or fresh peach instead of using jam on a peanut butter sandwich. Make your own fizzy drinks with unsweetened fruit juice and sparkling water.

Pass on the sugar: Take the sugar bowl off the table and, if you add sugar to your tea, gradually cut down until you need none at all. Persevere with this because once your taste buds get used to tea and other hot drinks without sugar, you'll never want to switch back. And while you are cutting down, reduce the amount of sugar you use in baking as well.

Don't ban sugar altogether: Some sugar, judiciously added to wholesome foods, may make them more appetising; a sprinkling of brown sugar on oatmeal or grapefruit, or a teaspoon of maple syrup on winter squash enhances the taste of these healthy options. It is better to avoid sugar substitutes, as some studies suggest that they can also have an adverse effect on your health.

Cereal killer: Some breakfast cereals have four or more teaspoons of sugar added to each serving! When you buy unsweetened cereals you may be saving money and you can add your own sweetener at home, if you choose. Sprinkle fresh, canned or dried fruit on your cereal to sweeten.

Read labels: When food shopping, read ingredient labels to find the amount and types of sugars that have been added to the food. There are many kinds of sugar that are used to make a food sweet and crisp. Look for words that end in 'ose' or 'ol', such as dextrose, fructose, maltose, sucrose, glucose, lactose, mannitol and sorbitol. These are all forms of sugar. Syrups such as corn sweetener, sorghum syrup and high-fructose syrups are sweeteners that are often added to drinks. Brown sugar, molasses and honey may be 'natural', but they all give you the same calories as refined table sugar. Ingredients are listed in order by weight, from most to least, so when a type of sugar or syrup is the first ingredient, you will know there is more sugar in that food than any other ingredient. Some foods may contain many kinds of sugar. When they are added up, the total may be more than any other ingredient in that food.

Switch from white bread, pasta and rice to wholegrain alternatives: Wholegrains are packed with nutrients and fibre that can keep your blood-sugar levels and your appetite balanced for hours after eating, unlike sugar, which gives you a quick high followed by a long low.

9 Conquer your sweet tooth

If you have a sweet tooth and constantly crave something sweet, you need to conquer it. A diet rich in sugar depresses your immune system and stops it working efficiently.

To conquer your sweet tooth, first of all, make sure you always eat breakfast and never leave more than two or three hours between meals and snacks. This is because eating little and often and kick-starting your metabolism first thing will keep your blood-sugar levels balanced so you are less likely to suffer from cravings. Aim for a healthy breakfast, followed by a satisfying mid-morning snack (a piece of fruit and a handful of nuts and seeds, for example), a healthy lunch, a mid-afternoon snack, supper and a light snack before bedtime.

For blood-sugar balance and appetite control, your meals and snacks need to be a mix of fibre-rich carbohydrates (such as wholegrains, fruits and vegetables) and healthy protein (such as nuts, seeds or dairy products) that give your body and brain a sustained release of energy so you feel satisfied. Avoid sweets, cakes, crisps and other processed or refined foods; these give you a quick burst of energy followed by a long, drawn-out low.

And finally, if cravings do strike, try these feisty, sweet treats. They'll satisfy your sweet tooth and boost your health and immunity at the same time:

A tablespoon or two of dried fruits: These are low in fat and have a low glycemic index, which means they're absorbed slowly from the stomach into the bloodstream and make you feel full for longer. Dried fruits are also high in immune- and energy-boosting iron and fibre.

Berry mix: In a large bowl, mix blueberries, raspberries, blackberries and cherries. This is a very healthy fruit snack. It's low in fat and contains a lot of vitamins and bioflavonoids that can boost immunity. You may also want to add some bone-building, calcium-rich low-fat natural yoghurt.

Fruit smoothie: A low-fat energy-boosting snack bursting with nutrients that tastes delicious (*see* pages 63 and 89).

10 Red, red wine

Treat yourself to a small glass of red wine with your meal. Recent studies show that drinking no more than one glass of red wine a day may have certain immune-boosting benefits by protecting against certain cancers and heart disease, and can have a positive effect on cholesterol levels and blood pressure.

Drinking wine with your meal, in addition to being good for your heart, may also help ward off food poisoning before it happens. Scientists at Oregon State University recently found that wine can put the kibosh on three common food pathogens: *E. coli*, listeria and salmonella. In lab studies, the wine's combination of ethanol and organic acids appeared to scramble the bugs' genetic material. All wines have a similar effect, say researchers, but reds are the most potent. Excessive or binge drinking, however, doesn't produce the same benefits.

Excessive alcohol intake can harm your body's immune system in two ways. First, it produces an overall nutritional deficiency, depriving the body of valuable immune-boosting nutrients. Second, alcohol, like sugar, consumed in excess can reduce the ability of white cells to kill germs. High doses of alcohol suppress the ability of the white blood cells to multiply, inhibit the action of killer white cells on cancer cells and lessen the ability of immune cells called macrophages to produce tumour necrosis factor, which kills cancer cells.

One drink (the equivalent of 350 ml (12 fl oz) of beer, 150 ml (5 fl oz) of wine, or 25 ml (1 fl oz) of spirits) does not appear to bother the immune system, but three or more drinks do. Damage to the immune system increases in proportion to the quantity of alcohol consumed, so, if you're tempted to buy another round, remember that amounts of alcohol that are enough to cause intoxication are also enough to suppress immunity.

11 Raw power

Cut down on the amount of
cooking you do, because
cooked food – especially
overcooked food – diminishes the amount of
immune-boosting nutrients.

This doesn't mean you shouldn't cook at all.
Certain foods such as eggs, meat and fish can be
dangerous to eat when raw, and need to be
cooked thoroughly. Try to balance cooked food
with raw food, perhaps 50:50, and cook gently,
at a lower heat and for longer if necessary. (It's
always best to avoid aluminium cookware as this
can increase the toxic load on your immune
system.) Steaming is the ideal way to cook
vegetables, stir-frying is a good way of cooking
fish, and poaching is useful for eggs and fish.
Meat should be roasted since other methods,
such as frying, use too much fat.

So, without going overboard, eat something
raw with every meal or begin each meal with
something raw – for example, an apple at
breakfast, and a stick of celery or some chopped
cucumber at lunch or supper.

12 Feel the burn

A curry once or twice a week can refresh your taste buds and your immune system.

Enjoying a curry every week or a dash or two of hot sauce with your meals could help keep bugs at bay. Several animal and laboratory studies have shown that capsaicin – the compound that gives chilli peppers their fire – can help stop sickness before it starts. In one study, mice were given a daily dose of capsaicin and had nearly three times more antibody-producing cells after three weeks than those given no capsaicin. More antibodies mean fewer colds and infections. Results of other studies suggest that eating food containing hot components such as capsaicin may improve immunity by flushing out toxins.

So if you like your food hot and spicy, go ahead and treat yourself. Curry is fast catching up with fish and chips as the UK's most popular takeaway – and as long as the ingredients used are fresh and additive free you'll be making a healthy choice.

13 Power-packed protein

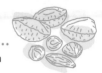

Savour some lean protein with every meal.

The amino acids found in protein form the building blocks of all the body's cells, including the cells that power your immune system. If you don't consume enough protein, you'll manufacture fewer white blood cells to combat disease-causing antigens.

One of the ways immune cells fight against pathogens is by increasing their own numbers; to stimulate immune cell proliferation, you need protein and amino acids. In addition, protein helps maintain blood-sugar balance and an immune-friendly alkaline state. Diets that are low in protein also tend to be high in carbohydrates, particularly refined carbohydrates, which convert readily to glucose, spiking blood sugar and stressing the pancreas and the immune system.

Your body can't store protein as it does carbohydrate and fat, so you need a constant supply; you should therefore try to eat some good-quality protein with every meal and snack. But remember that quality counts. To avoid the health risks of saturated fat, choose 75–125 g (3–4 oz) portions of lean protein such as fish, seafood, poultry (without the skin), eggs, lentils and pulses, and soy products. Other great sources of protein include dairy products, wheat germ, spirulina, grains such as quinoa, leafy green vegetables, peas, nuts, seeds, seaweed and Quorn.

Don't go overboard as a high protein diet can lead to an increased risk of diabetes and heart disease. That's why, as well as eating some protein with every meal and snack, you also need to eat nutritious and healthy carbohydrates and fats as part of a varied and balanced diet. Aim to get about 25 per cent of your total daily calorie intake from protein sources; 20–25 per cent from healthy fats and the rest from carbohydrates in the form of wholegrains, fruits and vegetables.

14 Go out of your whey

Sprinkle some immune-strengthening whey protein powder on your smoothies or yoghurts.

Whey protein offers an impressive range of benefits that most of us simply don't know about. Not only can whey protein boost weight loss and cardiovascular health, it can also support your immune system and boost bone mineral density.

Adding whey protein to your diet is a powerful way to boost your immunity. This is because whey protein is rich in an amino acid called cysteine, which converts to glutathione in the body. Glutathione is a potent antioxidant that fortifies cells against bacterial or viral infection. For the highest concentration of protein, try powdered whey protein isolate, which is more pure – and a little more expensive – than concentrate.

Fortify your morning smoothie with whey protein powder or try another source: live natural yoghurt. The clear liquid that forms on top of most yoghurt cartons is pure whey protein – so don't drain it off, just stir it back into the yoghurt.

Whey protein fruit smoothie

125 g (4 oz) live natural yoghurt
125–200 ml (4–7 fl oz) water
100 g (3½ oz) fresh or frozen berries
1 medium-sized banana
1 scoop whey protein powder
2 or 3 ice cubes (not needed if using frozen fruit)

Put all the ingredients in a blender and whizz until smooth.

Natural yoghurt with whey powder

1 scoop whey protein powder
125 g (4 oz) live natural yoghurt
½ tsp honey
Cinnamon sprinkles, to garnish

Stir whey protein powder into a bowl of live natural yoghurt. Add honey and top with cinnamon sprinkles.

15 Antioxidant protection on a plate

Stockpile antioxidant-rich
foods and your immune system
will grow stronger by the day.

Antioxidants are a group of vitamins,
minerals and unique compounds with incredible
immune-boosting benefits, protecting your cells
from free radical damage. Free radicals cause
cellular damage and can trigger disease, and
are produced by all kinds of combustion –
environmental pollution, smoking, radiation,
fried foods (high levels of heat damages the oil).
Fortunately, nature supplies us with rich sources
of antioxidant nutrients to disarm free radicals
and offers instant protection on a plate.

To protect against free radical damage,
your diet needs to be rich in the following
antioxidants: vitamin A, beta carotene,
vitamin C, vitamin E, zinc and selenium. Of all
these antioxidants, vitamin C is the king since it
is antibacterial as well as antiviral, and is a
natural antihistamine that helps with the body's
response to allergens. Eating six servings of fresh

fruit and vegetables each day will give you around 200 mg of vitamin C (the recommended daily amount). High-level sources of vitamin C include: citrus fruits, kiwi fruit, papaya, strawberries, blackcurrants, green vegetables, tomatoes, potatoes, broccoli, red and green peppers, and parsley.

To ensure you are getting enough antioxidant protection try to make your snacking fruitful, add more fruit and vegetables to your cooking, and get used to serving two vegetables with your meals instead of one. And don't forget that vegetable and fruit smoothies and juices count too.

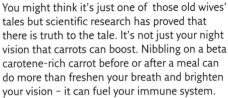

16 A carrot a day

Most of us grow up hearing 'eat up your carrots, they'll help you to see in the dark.' You might think it's just one of those old wives' tales but scientific research has proved that there is truth to the tale. It's not just your night vision that carrots can boost. Nibbling on a beta carotene-rich carrot before or after a meal can do more than freshen your breath and brighten your vision – it can fuel your immune system.

Studies have shown that the antioxidant beta carotene can lower the risk of cardiovascular disease, especially strokes and heart attacks, giving scientific support to the belief that a carrot a day can keep the heart surgeon away. Beta carotene also protects against cancer by stimulating the immune cells called macrophages to produce tumour necrosis factor, which kills cancer cells.

Beta carotene is present in yellow and orange fruits and vegetables such as carrots, tomatoes, mangoes, sweet potatoes, red and yellow peppers, and dark green vegetables such as spinach, watercress and broccoli.

Immune-boosting carrot soup

1 tbsp extra virgin olive oil
1 medium onion, chopped
7 large carrots, washed, peeled and chopped
2.5 cm (1 in) cube of fresh ginger root, chopped
1 vegetable stock cube
900 ml (1½ pints) boiling water
1 tsp freshly ground black pepper
1 tbsp fresh basil to garnish
Sea salt, to taste

1   Heat the oil in a large pan. Add the onion, carrots and ginger, and cook for five minutes to soften.
2   In a separate measuring cup, make up the vegetable stock using the boiling water and stock cube. Add to the pan and bring to the boil. Cover the saucepan and let simmer for 35 minutes or until the carrots are tender.
3   Pour the contents of the pan into a food processor or blender. Add the black pepper and blitz to a smooth consistency, adding more water if needed. You may have to do this in two batches.
4   Return the soup to the pan and warm through gently. Check the seasoning, then garnish with basil and serve.

17 Dress for success

The next time you order or prepare
a salad, add a generous portion of
olive or nut oil to your dressing.

Eating salad is a smart food
choice at lunch or dinner but dousing
it in fat-free dressing isn't. A study undertaken at
Iowa State University found that without dietary
fat, your body doesn't absorb some of the
disease-fighting nutrients in vegetables.
Researchers fed seven people salad for twelve
weeks and tested their blood after each meal.
Those who topped their salads with fat-free
dressing consistently failed to absorb
carotenoids (antioxidants that have been linked
to improved immunity).

Fat is necessary for the carotenoids to reach
the absorptive intestinal cells, so be sure to
choose dressings made with healthy fats such as
extra virgin olive oil, sunflower or flaxseed oil.
And if you're feeling adventuresome, try making
your own dressing. Don't just stick with tried and
tested olive oil. Experiment with other types of
healthy oil such as sunflower, sesame and nut oil.

18 Put SEZ on your plate

Vitamin C and vitamin A aren't the only antioxidants that boost your immunity. To get your full quota of antioxidant protection you need to ensure you put enough SEZ – selenium, vitamin E and zinc – on your plate every day.

- Selenium increases natural killer cells and mobilises cancer-fighting cells. Good food sources include nuts (especially Brazil nuts), seeds, wholegrains, seafood, egg yolks, sunflower seeds and garlic.
- Vitamin E increases the production of natural killer cells that hunt and destroy unwanted viruses, bacteria and cancer cells. Good food sources of vitamin E are avocados, nuts, seeds, unrefined oils and oatmeal.
- Zinc promotes the growth of immune-boosting white blood cells, especially the lymphocytes. Good food sources include lean meat, ginger, pumpkin seeds, Brazil nuts and wholegrains.

Snacking on some iron-rich dried fruits, such as raisins, during the day will give your immune system a kick-start.

Iron is a mineral that is needed for the production of white blood cells and antibodies, and without sufficient iron you are more likely to suffer from frequent colds and infections. A diet deficient in iron can also increase your risk of anaemia, a condition in which red blood cells are not providing adequate oxygen to body tissues and symptoms include fatigue, shortness of breath and bleeding gums. The best sources of dietary iron are lean red meat, seafood (such as lake trout, clams and oysters), eggs, legumes (such as beans, peas and lentils), nuts, seeds, wholegrains, dried fruits, green leafy vegetables and iron-enriched cereals and pastas.

Non-meat sources of iron are easier to absorb if combined with a good source of vitamin C, such as citrus fruit or juice, berries, peppers, broccoli, cabbage, tomatoes, Brussels sprouts, cantaloupe melons, kiwi fruits, mangoes and papayas.

Iron-rich vegetable juice recipe

1 glass filtered water
1 beetroot, washed and finely chopped
2 carrots, washed, peeled and finely chopped
2 tomatoes, washed, skinned and finely
  chopped
3 leaves fresh spinach, washed and finely
  chopped
Fresh lime or lemon juice to aid absorption
  (add a few drops first and then add more
  according to taste)
Pinch of black pepper

1 To make this healthy morning drink, put all
   the ingredients in a blender.
2 Cover and process until smooth.
   Serve immediately.

20 More omega-3s

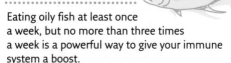

Eating oily fish at least once a week, but no more than three times a week is a powerful way to give your immune system a boost.

A high-fat diet can impair your immune system by decreasing the function of T-lymphocytes. Saturated fats (found in animal products and fried foods) can contribute to heart disease and weight gain, while transfats (found in margarines and many commercial baked goods) can contribute to chronic low-grade inflammation in the body. So limit consumption of fat to 30 per cent of your daily calorie intake, with 5–10 per cent from saturated fats. For the remaining 20–25 per cent, look for sources of unsaturated fats, such as canola oil, olive oil, nuts, avocados and seeds. And increase your intake of omega-3 fatty acids, which help fight inflammation and free your immune system to defend against antigens.

Well-documented for their ability to protect us from heart disease, omega-3 fatty acids are found in oily fish such as mackerel, sardines, salmon, trout and fresh (but not tinned) tuna. They help immunity by stimulating the activity of white blood cells that attack bacteria.

A recent study found that children taking half a teaspoon of flax oil a day experienced fewer and less severe respiratory infections, as well as fewer days' absence from school. The omega-3 fatty acids in flax oil and oily fish act as immune boosters by increasing the activity of phagocytes, the white blood cells that eat up bacteria. (Perhaps this is why grandmothers used to insist on a daily dose of unpalatable cod liver oil.) Essential fatty acids also protect the body against damage from over-reactions to infection.

If you're vegetarian or don't like fish, you can increase your intake of this micro-nutrient by incorporating flax oil into your diet. One simple way to get more omega-3 fatty acids in your diet is to add 1–3 teaspoons of flax oil to a fruit-and-yoghurt smoothie, or to salads or other dishes. The oil loses nutrients when heated, so it is best eaten cold.

21 Maintain an energy balance

Your immune system works best when you eat enough – neither too many nor too few – calories per day.

Over-consumption of calories can have harmful effects on cell production in the immune system by increasing the production of compounds called prostaglandins, which have a suppressive effect on T-lymphocyte cell production. Fewer T cells patrolling the body increases the chances of an antigen taking hold.

On the other hand, under-consumption of calories can be just as harmful. Considerable evidence shows crash dieting, anorexia or nutrient deficiencies increase a person's susceptibility to infections. Going on a low-calorie diet or going for long periods without food is one sure-fire way to lower your immunity. This is because if you starve yourself, your body will think it's under siege and pump out stress hormones that both unsettle your blood-sugar levels and have a damaging impact on your immunity. In addition, losing more than 1 kg (2.2 lb) per week is hard on the T cells that detect diseased or foreign cells.

Studies have shown that the best and most effective way to lose weight, if you have weight to lose, is to lose it gradually. A 2007 study at the University of California – to date, the world's largest investigation into weight loss – showed that dieting is damaging because of dieters' tendency to lose and then regain weight; this yo-yo dieting effect increases the risk of heart attacks, strokes and diabetes. Starving yourself or depriving your body of the nutrients it needs to boost your immunity and metabolism (fat burning) will therefore not only increase your likelihood of succumbing to a cold or flu – it will also almost inevitably lead you to piling your weight straight back on.

Being overweight can weaken your immunity, but don't try and remedy this by going on a strict diet as this could make things worse. If you have weight to lose, aim for a loss of no more than ½–1 kg (1–2 lb) a week, and maintain that vital energy balance by eating healthily and increasing the amount of exercise you do.

22 Eggs is easy

Having an egg for breakfast every day is a great way to boost your energy levels and to make sure you get a fix of immune-boosting magnesium.

You've probably heard a great deal about the importance of calcium for building healthy, strong bones but less about the importance of eating enough foods rich in its immune-boosting partner, magnesium.

Magnesium is required for antibody protection and low magnesium levels can increase the risk of allergic reactions because a magnesium deficiency can cause histamine levels to rise. Good food sources include nuts, seeds, green leafy vegetables, root vegetables, egg yolks, wholegrains and dried fruit.

Not only are calcium and magnesium important for boosting immunity, they also can't work well without each other. This is because magnesium helps your body absorb calcium, so even if your diet is rich in calcium you can still be deficient if you aren't eating enough magnesium-rich foods.

23 Put the kettle on

Every time you put your feet up and enjoy a cup of tea, your immune system gets a natural boost.

Many studies support the view that tea is good for your health. Scientists tend to agree that tea, both black and green, may contribute positively to the promotion of health and the prevention of chronic disease. Recent research has revealed that the antioxidants in tea may inhibit the growth of cancerous cells, support dental health, increase bone density and strengthen cardiovascular health.

According to a recent study, heart attack patients who were tea drinkers decreased their risk of death by up to 44 per cent when compared with non-tea drinkers and there was no evidence that tea was dehydrating or that consumption of three or four cups a day was harmful to health. In fact they positively recommended it.

Research, however, does suggest that tea can impair the body's ability to absorb iron from food, indicating that people at risk of anaemia should avoid drinking tea around mealtimes.

24 The magic of garlic

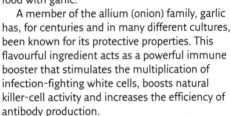

Add a touch of immune-
boosting magic to your diet
by cooking or preparing your
food with garlic.

A member of the allium (onion) family, garlic
has, for centuries and in many different cultures,
been known for its protective properties. This
flavourful ingredient acts as a powerful immune
booster that stimulates the multiplication of
infection-fighting white cells, boosts natural
killer-cell activity and increases the efficiency of
antibody production.

The immune-boosting properties of garlic
seem to be due to its sulphur-containing
compounds, such as allicin and sulfides, which
provide garlic with its distinctive taste. Garlic
also acts as an antioxidant that reduces the
build-up of free radicals in the bloodstream and
plays a part in getting rid of potential carcino-
gens and other toxic substances; evidence for
this can be found in the fact that cultures with a
garlic-rich diet have a lower incidence of
intestinal cancer. It is also a heart-friendly food

since it keeps platelets from sticking together and clogging tiny blood vessels.

Crush garlic into stews, roast it alongside meat or mash it with avocado and lemon juice to make an immune-system-friendly stew. If you don't like the taste of garlic (or are worried about garlic-smelling breath), try the odourless and flavourless supplements in capsule form that are now available in health food stores.

Garlic bread

1 loaf French bread
(125 g) 4 oz butter, unsalted
(50 g) 2 oz fresh parsley, finely chopped
2 large garlic cloves, crushed and chopped finely
Paprika (optional)

1 Cut bread into 2.5 cm (1-inch) thick slices, but not all the way through.
2 Combine butter, parsley and garlic, mixing well.
3 Spread between bread slices and sprinkle with paprika, if desired.
4 Reassemble the loaf, wrap in foil and bake for 20 minutes at 180°C (350°F) Gas 4.

25 Green leafy defence

Green leafy vegetables, such as broccoli, kale and spinach, are packed with immune-boosting, cancer-fighting antioxidant power. Be sure to eat your greens every day or every other day.

Spinach is rich in carotenoids, which the body converts to vitamin A to help trigger the immune response. The vitamin C content of spinach keeps skin and mucous membranes healthy, while its vitamin B content boosts energy. Spinach is also an excellent source of zinc, which is required to promote T cell activity. Try this warming immune-boosting dish.

Spinach and potato bake

300 g (11 oz) spinach
150 g (5 oz) crème fraîche
2 tbsp grainy mustard
1 garlic clove, crushed
750 g (1½ lb) potatoes, peeled and
thinly sliced

1 Lightly steam the spinach, drain well and chop finely.
2 Mix the crème fraîche with the mustard and the crushed clove of garlic.
3 Use a third of the potato to cover the base of an ovenproof dish, then place half the spinach on top of the potato and pour over some of the crème fraîche mixture.
4 Add another layer of each, finishing with a layer of potato and crème fraîche mixture.
5 Cover with foil and bake for one hour at 180°C (350°F) Gas 4.
6 Remove the foil and bake for a further 20 minutes or until tender and lightly brown.

26 Brilliant berries

All berries are brilliant for immunity boosting because they are power-packed with vitamin C, but blackcurrants and blueberries in particular stand out.

Blackcurrants contain nutrients that can improve iron absorption, boost metabolism and enhance oxygen transport to the tissues. They aid liver function, help regulate blood-sugar levels and encourage wound healing. They may also offer protection against heart disease and cancer.

Blueberries are one of the richest sources of immune-boosting, cancer-fighting, anti-ageing antioxidants you can eat, and scientists have discovered that they possess many other health benefits, such as improving brain function and balancing blood-sugar levels. Try this immune-boosting berry smoothie, which also contains apple (apples contain pectin, which has cancer-fighting properties; they are also packed with vitamin C, calcium, magnesium and beta carotene, and can help flush out your liver and kidneys):

Brilliant berry smoothie

1 large apple
150 ml (5 fl oz) natural live yoghurt
8 blackberries
8 blueberries
8 raspberries
Handful of organic porridge oats
1 tsp maple syrup (optional)

1 Juice the apple, then place with the yoghurt
   in a blender.
2 Add the berries and blend until smooth.
3 Pour into a shallow glass and sprinkle the oats
   on top, with an optional drizzle of maple syrup
   over the oats.
4 For a swirl effect, keep back half the yoghurt
   and gently stir it in after blending until a
   marbled effect is achieved.

To give your immune system a lift, slice some avocado into your sandwiches and salads.

Avocado is packed with energy and immune-boosting phytochemicals that can help protect against certain cancers. A rich source of skin-friendly antioxidants, it also helps stabilise blood sugar and blood pressure, and is a good source of vitamin C, and vitamin E and B6.

Avocado salad

> 2 avocados
> romaine lettuce leaves
> ½ tsp black pepper
> 1/2 tsp dried oregano
> 1 garlic clove, chopped
> 1 sprig fresh thyme
> 4–5 tbsp extra virgin olive oil
> 1 tbsp red wine; 1 tbsp vinegar

1 Cut the avocados in half and discard the stone. Scoop out the avocado flesh with an ice cream scoop and shape into little balls. Place them on two plates lined with the lettuce leaves.
2 In a small bowl, whisk together the rest of the ingredients, pour over the avocados and serve.

28 See red

Tomatoes are packed with antioxidants including vitamins A
and C, together with lycopene,
which can improve your immune response,
boost resistance to infectious disease, encourage
wound healing and keep the skin and muscles in
good condition. In a study published in the
American Journal of Clinical Nutrition, ten
subjects ate a tomato-rich diet for three weeks,
followed by a tomato-free diet for three more
weeks. While subjects were on the tomato diet,
their infection-fighting white blood cells sustained
38 per cent less damage from free radicals –
atoms in the body that damage and destabilise
cells – than when they ate no tomato products.

Researchers speculate that the lycopene in
tomatoes acts as an antioxidant, helping white
blood cells resist the damaging effects of free
radicals. Try baked tomatoes (or beans and
tomatoes) on wholegrain toast, as well as
homemade tomato soup. And don't forget that
tomato ketchup – if used in moderation, is also a
source of immune-boosting lycopene.

29 Instant protection

Every time you include the following foods in your food or cooking you give your immune defences an instant pick-me-up.

Cinnamon: This culinary spice has wonderful antibacterial and antifungal properties. To make yourself a warm toddy, fill a cup with boiling water and add two teaspoons of tea-tree honey, the juice of a lemon and one quarter of a cinnamon stick. Allow the drink to steep for 10 minutes and then remove the cinnamon stick; relax and enjoy.

Nuts and seeds: A handful of nuts and seeds as a between-meal snack or sprinkled on your salad or soup will give your immune system a welcome shot of protein, zinc, B vitamins, vitamin E, selenium, magnesium and essential fats. Brazil nuts are a wonderful source of selenium. Almonds, hazelnuts and sunflower seeds are best for vitamin E, while flaxseeds are great for omega-3, sunflower seeds for omega-6, protein and B vitamins, and pumpkin seeds are an especially good source of zinc, which is needed for healthy skin and white blood cell function.

Parsley power: Parsley is a must for every refrigerator or windowbox because it is rich in vitamins A and C, as well as magnesium and cancer-fighting chlorophyll.

Seaweed: A wealth of minerals, vitamins and amino acids can be found in seaweed, so try adding a little to your soups or mix with mashed potato.

Shiitake mushrooms: Great in stews, soups and stir-fries, shiitake mushrooms possess antibacterial, antiviral and anti-parasitic properties and are a natural source of protection against viruses.

Sweet potato: A rich source of vitamin E, sweet potato can contribute to heart health and is a good source of dietary antioxidants. It can help to regulate high blood pressure, and its vitamin A and carotenoid content may offer protection against inflammatory conditions. Why not give sweet potato mash or sweet potato curry a try?

30 Brighter breakfast smoothie

Give your immune system and your health an energy shot first thing in the morning with this bright and energising smoothie.

This tropical fruit smoothie is just the thing to help boost your immune system. Few people are aware of the high levels of vitamin C that are found in kiwi fruit. In fact, weight for weight, the kiwi fruit contains twice as much vitamin C as oranges. They are also a good source of potassium, which can help to maintain a healthy heart. Mangoes are a good source of vitamin C and carotenoids, both of which help to strengthen the immune system. The smoothness of the coconut milk helps to balance the tartness of the kiwi fruit. Spirulina is a nutrition-packed blue-green algae seaweed that can strengthen your immune system. It has gained prominence as nature's green 'superfood' because of its rich concentration of perfectly balanced amino acids (protein), fibre, vitamins, minerals and other essential nutrients.

Breakfast smoothie

2 kiwi fruit, peeled and chopped
1 mango or 1 nectarine, peeled chopped and
destoned
100 ml (3½ fl oz) coconut milk
2 tsp spirulina powder
75 ml (3 fl oz) live natural yoghurt
2 tsp maple syrup (optional, to taste)
Ice cubes, to serve

1 Place the roughly chopped kiwi and mango in
   your blender or smoothie maker along with the
   coconut milk.
2 Blend until the large fruit chunks start to
   disappear and then add the spirulina powder,
   yoghurt and maple syrup, if liked; continue
   blending until smooth.
3 Serve over ice and enjoy pronto!

31 Bon appétit!

Every time you sit down and really savour every mouthful of your food, you are – believe it or not – boosting your immunity.

Most people think that digestion begins in the stomach but the process actually begins in the mouth. Taking time to sit down and chew your food properly allows your saliva to alkalise it (remember, bacteria prefer an acid environment) and stimulates the production of essential, digestive enzymes. The process of chewing is a vital component of the digestive activities that occur in the mouth, being inextricably linked to good digestion, and therefore, good health and immunity.

Taking time to enjoy your food isn't as easy as it sounds – most of us rush our meals and gulp food more than we realise. In order to get the maximum immune-boosting nutritional benefit from your food you need to slow down and chew it thoroughly. So don't eat at your desk and don't try to grab a bite to eat as you run from one appointment to another. Set aside the time to ensure that the food you eat is a proper meal rather than simply fuel you need to take on board as quickly as possible.

The next time you have a meal or snack, concentrate on noticing every morsel; how does it look, smell and taste. Count to five between each bite or put your knife and fork down between bites. In reality it doesn't really take much time and effort to chew your food, and what you get in return is better digestion, better health and stronger immunity, as well as a greater enjoyment of your food. Chewing and savouring your food is important but also make sure that you eat in a calm and peaceful environment. Avoid distractions that make you more likely to overeat or mindlessly shovel food into your mouth. Turn off the television and try not to read or work as you eat.

Boosting immunity with lifestyle changes

32 Douse the night light

Keep your bedroom as dark as possible when you are sleeping. Too much brightness during the night depresses your immune system.

Only when it's really dark does your body produce melatonin, a hormone that not only helps you drift off to sleep but also helps prevent certain diseases.

Even a dim source such as a bedside clock or a night light may switch melatonin production off, so keep your bedroom as dark as possible. And if light from street lamps shines into your bedroom, invest in some black-out curtains.

33 Get a full night's sleep

Everyone is different – your body may need anywhere from 6–8 hours of sleep each night. Whatever your personal sleep requirement is, make sure you get it!

Sleeping better may help you fight off illness. People who are sleep-deprived often have raised levels of stress hormones, as well as running the risk of persistent inflammation in the blood and a decrease in immune function.

Quality sleep has been linked to balanced hormone levels (including human growth hormone and the stress hormone cortisol); these keep weight down, lead to clear thinking and reasoning, improve mood and engender vibrant, healthy skin. New research from a Warwick study of the sleep patterns of some 10,000 Britons links cutting sleep to five hours or fewer to a doubled risk of dying from cardio-vascular disease. Shortage of sleep is also linked to increased risk of weight gain and diabetes.

Put simply, people who sleep well live longer. So if you want good health and to live to a ripe old age, get an early night.

34 Pick up the pace

Walking at a brisk pace every
day for 20-30 minutes
stimulates the production of a
variety of immune cells and
enhances the overall function of the
immune system.

Researchers from the University of South
Carolina and the University of Massachusetts
recently studied 550 adults. Those who simply
walked at a brisk pace had about 25 per cent fewer
colds than those who seldom or never exercised.
Results of at least three clinical trials tend to
confirm this finding. In all three trials, women
who were told to walk briskly most days over a
three-month period developed colds only about
half as often as those who did no exercise at all.

The research shows that during moderate
exercise, several positive changes occur in the
immune system. Various immune cells circulate
through the body more quickly and are better
able to kill bacteria and viruses. Once the
exercise session is over, the immune system
returns to normal. The preliminary conclusions

are that moderate exercise, such as a brisk walk, will give your immune system a boost, and this in turn should increase your chances of fighting off cold viruses in the long term.

Exercise that increases your heart rate and moves large muscles (such as those in your legs and arms) is what you should aim for. Choose an activity that you enjoy and can start slowly; gradually, as you get fitter, aim to work out for 20–30 minutes four to six times a week. Walking briskly is very popular and does not require any special equipment or training. Other good exercises if you feel more energetic include swimming, cycling, gentle jogging and tram-polining. Even if you are pushed for time, benefits can be gained simply by walking upstairs rather than taking the lift, or by walking or cycling on shorter journeys rather than taking the car.

35 Pick a fight

Sign up for a martial arts class
or some basic instruction in
the art of wrestling and see
your health and fitness improve.

One study put 11 healthy boys aged
between 14 and 18 through a 90-minute
wrestling practice session, sampling their blood
before and after the session. The study found
that levels of all groups of white blood cells,
particularly the natural killer cells, rose
significantly. The killer cells fight cancer and
viruses by searching out the equivalent of a
flag carried by normal cells. Those without
such a flag are attacked by a cocktail of
chemicals.

Another study, this time on martial arts,
compared the fitness levels of nine people aged
between 40 and 60 who practised Soo bahk do
(a martial art similar to karate) with those of nine
sedentary people. Those who did the martial art
were found to have better levels of body fat,
balance, flexibility, muscle strength, endurance
and aerobic capacity.

Martial arts – even mild forms like T'ai chi – have long been known to confer tremendous immune-boosting anti-aging health benefits to their followers. Throughout Asia, it's not uncommon to see large groups of elderly (people in their sixties, seventies and eighties) practising T'ai chi at sunrise in community parks. Despite their age, these people have better aerobic conditioning, balance, strength, flexibility and coordination than many typical Westerners in their thirties. Any form of martial arts will produce similar benefits. In addition to T'ai chi, the more combative kick boxing and Tae kwon do are also excellent, but do make sure you sign up for a beginners class and get the okay from your GP if you are on medication or suffering from a medical condition.

36 Take to the floor

Join a dance class or put some music on and dance around your living room. Half an hour of gentle dancing is equivalent to the same length of time of brisk walking in terms of calorie consumption, while more energetic forms of dance, such as disco and rock'n'roll, will burn even more.

Experts recommend that we all do 30 minutes of moderate aerobic activity most days of the week for heart health and for keeping colds and bugs at bay. Dance uses oxygen, burns calories and increases your heart's workload, so it's ideal. Dance also has many advantages over more standard forms of exercise. You can set your own pace: a slow foxtrot is no more energetic than walking, while a salsa will really get your heart pumping. It's great fun too, and an excellent way to meet people, which means that it will never become a bore or a chore.

A study carried out in Denmark of men and women aged 60 to 82 who were healthy but did not exercise found that, in as little as five months, regular dancing markedly improved levels of unhealthy blood fats associated with furring of the arteries. US research shows that a vigorous dance class or disco session can burn as many calories as a gym workout.

Dance combines aerobic activity with weight-bearing exercise, which will boost your strength and endurance. One woman in four and one man in eight is at risk of the brittle bone disease osteoporosis. Dancing slightly jars the bones, thereby encouraging the body to build new bone and helps strengthen the skeleton. And finally, in common with any sustained aerobic activity, dance releases endorphins, which are body-made chemicals that ease pain, help banish depression and encourage feelings of well-being.

37 Workout, but don't overdo it

If you aren't an athlete or professional dancer, and are exercising for over an hour a day several times a week, give yourself and your immune cells a break and cut down on your work out time.

As with diet, moderation is crucial; too much exercise or exercising to the point of exhaustion can boost the body's production of adrenaline and cortisol – two hormones that temporarily suppress immune function. Olympians and other highly trained athletes often report that after intense competition and training they are more susceptible to colds. The exercise slogan of the 1980s, 'no pain, no gain', has fortunately given way to a more realistic notion that moderate exercise confers more health benefits than strenuous exercise. Moderate exercisers have the added benefit of suffering fewer injuries as well.

Exercising too hard and for too long isn't good for your immune system, so you need to aim for moderate exercise. One way to ensure that you are exercising at the right pace is to see if you can carry on a conversation while you are exercising. You should be slightly out of breath but not panting and unable to speak. So if you find yourself panting, huffing and puffing, STOP! You're exercising too hard.

While intensive training is what some prefer, rest assured that something as simple as a 30-minute daily walk will provide your body with all the health and immune benefits it needs. The key is, no matter how you get your exercise, to do it regularly and make sure it's fun!

38 Lose the baggage

Losing a little extra weight will not only reduce your risk of cardiovascular disease and diabetes, but will also help shape up your immune system.

Being excessively thin is associated with poor immunity because it means a person isn't getting the nutritional defences he or she needs to fight disease. But being too heavy for your height and build is also associated with impaired immune responses. Researchers at Tufts University asked a group of slightly overweight people to cut 100–200 calories from their daily food intake. In addition to weight loss, the results also showed that participants boosted their immune system response to disease-causing micro-organisms.

Researchers aren't exactly sure why weight loss – if you have weight to lose – is so beneficial, but speculate that the benefit comes from a combination of effects. One thing is certain: if you know you need to lose weight, losing that extra baggage (even if it is just a few pounds) will give your health and immunity a significant boost.

To lose weight safely, make sure that you eat five or six meals and snacks a day to keep your blood-sugar levels and your appetite steady; go for fresh, wholesome foods and ditch processed, refined foods. In addition, watch your portion size and make sure you eat plenty of fibre-rich wholegrains and immune-boosting fruits and vegetables. Start by cutting 200 calories out of your daily diet. At your next restaurant meal, ditch the baked potato with sour cream and order steamed vegetables instead. At snack time, reach for some fruit and a handful of nuts and seeds instead of the biscuits; and double up on vegetables instead of chips. Finally, step up the exercise. Most weight-loss experts recommend 30–40 minutes of physical activity a day for weight loss. Also try adding weight-bearing exercises at least two times a week. This will help build muscle mass and burn off more unwanted calories.

39 Work up a sweat

Work up a sweat, even if the barometer drops. Perspiration is a great way to remove toxins and other infection-friendly waste material from your body.

Have you noticed how, when you get an infection, you also get a fever or the local area becomes hot? An increase in body temperature is your immune system's way of actively fighting infection and disease. Sweating promotes the release of stored toxins through your skin, easing the toxic load on your body.

You can work up a sweat through exercise or when you do everyday tasks, such as gardening or housework. Using a sauna can also provide benefits, but if you do have a medical condition check with your doctor first before exposing yourself to high temperatures. You don't need to be saturated with perspiration. Remember that overdoing exercise is not immune-system friendly – a gentle sweat will do your immune system a power of good, bringing a rosy glow to your cheeks at the same time.

But what if it's too late and you haven't managed to avoid that cold? Should you rest or try to sweat it out? Much depends on your symptoms. In general, if your symptoms are above your neck and you have no fever, gentle exercise or building up a light sweat is probably safe. Intensive exercise should be postponed until after the symptoms have gone away. However, if there are symptoms and signs of flu, such as fever or swollen glands, at least ten days should be set aside before you resume ordinary training.

40 Cold shower burst

Turning the water to cold for a minute or so at the end of your shower stimulates lymphatic circulation that transports immune cells around your body.

Even though it may sound like a masochistic act, taking cold showers to reap health benefits isn't a new concept; it has been used as a means of therapy for thousands of years. The ancient art of yoga, which began an estimated four to eight thousand years ago, teaches its students that taking cold water showers will help strengthen their immune system against colds and flu. The theory is that coldness can help bring blood to the capillaries, therefore increasing circulation throughout the body. It also encourages muscles to contract so that toxins and poisonous waste can be eliminated more efficiently, painful inflammations are reduced and the mucous membranes are strengthened, which in turn helps keep hay fever, allergies, colds and coughs at bay. Some experts believe that many health problems can be reduced or even eliminated over time by providing proper circulation of the blood to the affected area using cold shower therapy.

There is no doubt that an invigorating way to enhance cleansing and to boost your circulation and immune system is to take a cold shower every day. Caution, however, is advised, especially if you are underweight or have a heart condition, as cold showers can put unnecessary stress on your heart. It's much safer and much more pleasant to have a warm shower first and then, just as you have finished soaping yourself or washing your hair and are ready to get out of the shower, to give yourself a cold shower burst for a minute. Make sure the bathroom is heated. Never get out of a cold shower into a cold room.

41 Take a breather

Deep breathing – from your abdomen not your lungs – can not only be relaxing, it can also raise your immunity.

Research on the link between oxygen deficiency and disease has been carried out for several decades, since oxygen plays a key role in our immune function. It is the source of ammunition used by killer and natural killer T cells against viruses and tumours. Breathing serves as the pump for the lymphatic system, just as the heart serves as the pump for the circulatory system. Your cells must have oxygen to survive from moment to moment. To thrive, they rely on a complex exchange between the circulatory system and the lymphatic system. Blood flow carries nutrients and ample amounts of oxygen into the capillaries, while a healthy lymphatic system carries away destructive toxins. Proper breathing is the moderator of this exchange.

Many of us breathe too fast and too rapidly during the day. This fast, shallow breathing expels carbon dioxide too quickly and takes in too little oxygen. However, when breathing is slow, deep and full – and is carried out from the abdomen (belly) and not the lungs – extra oxygen is drawn into the bloodstream. Your diaphragm is a thick, flat muscle just below your ribcage and above your abdomen. By using your diaphragm when you breathe in, you help your lungs expand so that they take in more air. Increased oxygenation boosts circulation and encourages the healthy functioning of your entire immune system.

Breathing from your diaphragm
1 Relax your shoulders and place one hand on your abdomen.
2 Breathe out and push your abdominal muscles out as you do so.
3 Breathe in through your nose and suck in your abdominal muscles.
4 Breathe out through your mouth with pursed lips (you should feel your abdomen go down).
5 Repeat three times and rest for two minutes. Repeat several times a day.

42 Rise and shine

Most of us relish the thought of a long lie-in, but that lie-in may be doing you more harm than good. It's far better to get up when you wake naturally.

A 2002 study found that getting more than seven hours of sleep each night was associated with a shorter life span.

Several subsequent studies, including one in 2006 by researchers at Brigham and Women's Hospital in Boston, also found a similar link, so it seems that – contrary to popular opinion – too much sleep can be as unhealthy and draining as too little. Sleep experts believe that between six and eight hours sleep a night is optimum for most people, which is less than was previously thought necessary. But whatever amount of sleep you need, if you want to wake up feeling refreshed and enjoy maximum health and vitality, your sleep must be regular. This means getting up and going to bed at the same time each day, including weekends. If you feel that you need to catch up on your sleep, avoid symptoms of jet lag without the holiday by going to bed earlier but still getting up at the same time.

43 Purse your lips
. . . .

Aerobic exercise is one way to
increase your intake of oxygen
and improve its circulation,
but immune-boosting benefits may also be
obtained from breathing exercises that teach
you to breathe more fully.

The following exercises will help you take
control of your breathing. These don't require a
lot of time, but work best if you commit to
practising a few minutes every day. Over time,
you will find that you are breathing more deeply
throughout the day and reaping all the immune-
boosting benefits. With practice, you can break
the cycle of bad breathing.

> **Hold your breath exercise**
> 1 Breathe in. Try to hold your breath for
>   ten seconds.
> 2 Breathe out with pursed lips as above.
> 3 Repeat three times.

Holding your breath extends the time your lungs can exchange oxygen for carbon dioxide, helping your body take in more oxygen.

Pursed-lip breathing exercise

1 Inhale slowly through your nose until your lungs fill up with air.
2 Purse your lips as if you were going to whistle or kiss someone. Breathe out slowly while keeping your lips pursed. Take twice as long to breathe out as you do to breathe in.
3 Do not force your lungs to empty.
4 Repeat five to six times.

Pursed-lip breathing will help you get more air into your lungs, encourage you to breathe more steadily and control any shortness of breath.

Three-part breathing exercise

1 With your mouth closed, exhale deeply through your nose. Imagine that you are pouring the breath out of a jug, starting at the top of your chest and moving down through your mid-torso and into your diaphragm.

2 Pause for two counts at the bottom of the breath and then inhale through your nose. Refill the jug slowly, counting to five (or seven if you can make it). Start at the bottom, expanding your diaphragm and belly, then your mid-torso, and lastly the top of your chest and lungs.

3 Pause for two counts and exhale as before. Then repeat the exercise three times.

This yoga technique is very useful during times of stress or any time you need to relax.

44 Snowball fight, anyone?

Most of us spend 90 per cent of our lives indoors inhaling dubiously filtered air and other people's germs, so take any opportunity you can to get some fresh air.

A regular dose of fresh air can help make your body less vulnerable to cold and flu viruses. This is especially true during cold weather when not only does central heating dehydrate you, but the tendency to stay indoors results in more germs circulating in crowded, dry rooms.

So even if it's cold outside, wrap up warm (*see* page 116) and get some energising fresh air. Go for a walk, have a gentle snowball fight or put your umbrella up and stroll in the rain. It's probably best to stay away from polluted areas and to seek out places where traffic is lighter and where there are signs of nature as the air is likely to be much fresher. Head to the countryside, seaside or the mountains if you can and, if you live or work in the city, seek out local parks, riverside paths and public gardens.

45 Take your sunglasses off

Even on cloudy days when the sun seems hidden, a daily dose of natural daylight provides you with a mood-boosting shot of vitamin D, an essential vitamin for healthy bones, a strong and hardy immune system and a good night's sleep.

Make sure you get at least 20–30 minutes of natural daylight every day, preferably without your sunglasses, glasses or lenses on, because you get most of your vitamin D from sunlight through your eyes. If it's a very hot day, wear sunscreen and avoid looking directly at the sun. And when you're outside remember to breathe deeply. This helps the lymphatic system to move your protective immune cells around the body.

Good dietary sources of vitamin D are eggs, liver, fish liver oils and oily fish such as salmon, sardines, trout and fresh (not tinned) tuna. But by far the best source of vitamin D is through sun exposure. When your skin is exposed to ultraviolet light, your body starts to manufacture vitamin D.

46 Keep your feet warm

To give yourself the best
chance of keeping healthy when
it's cold, wrap up before you go
out, remembering to keep your hands,
head, nose and – especially – your feet warm
and cosy.

Folklore suggests that chilling the surface of
the body through wet clothes, feet and hair
causes common cold symptoms to develop; but
past research has dismissed the relationship
between chilling and viral infection as having no
scientific basis. In 2005, however, researchers
from Cardiff University – with the aid of bowls of
ice water and people's feet – appear to have
shown that this is one piece of folklore that may
indeed be true: being chilly really can encourage
a cold to develop.

We get more winter illnesses in Britain than
in any other country in Europe. The reason for
this may be that we under-dress. Researchers
visiting European cities found that when the
temperature drops, people put on hats, scarves,
gloves and anoraks. We don't. We stand around

shivering waiting for buses and trains, and that is really bad news. If you have reached the shivering stage, your core temperature has dropped so much that your body believes it's an emergency. The blood gets much thicker, which causes heart attacks and strokes, and the immune system is weakened, so you pick up bugs more easily.

It's important to point out that although exposure to cold and damp weather may hamper the immune function of the respiratory system, if there is no exposure to a virus, then it's virtually impossible to get a cold. However, if you are cold and damp and come into contact with a virus, your risk of catching an infection is higher. So to give yourself the best chance of keeping healthy when it's cold outside, wrap up warm. And put on an extra pair of socks. According to the Common Cold Research Centre, cold feet lower the effective-ness of the immune system and enable viruses to flourish. It might also be a good idea to wear socks to bed, as research also shows that warm feet increase your chances of a good night's sleep.

47 Give your skin a brush

Dry skin brushing is another way to stimulate your lymphatic system and boost your immunity.

Your lymphatic system is a network of tiny fluid vessels throughout your body that transport toxins, bacteria, viruses and dead cells to lymph nodes. It's the job of your lymph nodes to break down, deactivate and purify these waste products so they are more easily handled by the organs of elimination, the liver and kidneys. A milky white fluid called lymph carries impurities and waste away from the tissues, and passes through gland-like structures spaced throughout the lymphatic system that act as filtering valves. The lymph does not circulate in the same way as the blood does, so its movement depends largely on the squeezing effect of muscle contractions. That's why exercise is so great for stimulating lymph flow.

When your lymph isn't circulating efficiently, you're more likely to succumb to infection and feel unwell. You're also more likely to have dark circles under your eyes, puffiness and a pale complexion (all signs of a sluggish lymphatic system). Exercise is the most effective way to stimulate the passage of lymph through the nodes, but it can also be stimulated through dry skin brushing.

The skin is your body's largest organ and when it functions efficiently, it eliminates almost a kilo of waste acids daily, so its ability to excrete toxins is crucial. When the skin ceases to function properly, an increased burden is placed on the lymphatic system and other excretory organs. Dry skin brushing removes the top layer of skin, which helps the skin excrete toxins and other acids in the body.

Dry brushing technique

The technique for dry skin brushing is simple and easy to do for a few minutes every morning. With a long-handled, firm, natural bristle bath brush, beginning at the soles of the feet and working your way up the legs, torso, back, hands and arms (in a circular motion and always towards the heart), brush away the dry, top layer of dead skin.

48 Rinse, don't soak

Rinsing rather than soaking fresh fruits and vegetables is an effective way to remove immune-suppressing pesticide residues.

Pesticides are chemicals used to protect crops from bugs, fungi, rodents and bacteria. If you use pesticides to rid your house of rodents or in the garden to remove weeds or insect blight then you, too, can be exposed to their dangerous effects. Pesticides may also be found in some plastics, household products and industrial chemicals. Animal and lab research suggests that these substances – which are potent, extremely toxic chemicals – damage your health, especially in high doses or with extended exposure, and may also degrade immune function. Other studies have found that people who work with pesticides may have weakened defences.

Although you are exposed to pesticides every day, thankfully there are things you can do to protect yourself:

- Rinse and gently scrub, but don't soak fresh fruits and vegetables.
- Trim the fat from meats. Some pesticides collect in animal fat.
- Peel fruits and vegetables before using them. Remove and discard the outer leaves of cabbages and other greens. If you buy organic, you need only scrub the skins.
- Eat a wide variety of fruits and vegetables, as specific pesticides are used for specific crops. This way you'll avoid eating too much of one specific pesticide.
- Use home, lawn and garden pesticides sparingly.
- Consider buying organic produce when it's available and affordable. Not only is organic produce pesticide-free, it will also be free of additives, preservatives, food colourings and other toxins that place a burden on your immune system. If you think organic produce is too expensive, consider buying just one item a week to get you into the habit of looking at it as an investment in your health. Specifically look for organically grown spinach, peaches, peppers, strawberries, apples, cherries, celery, apricots, green beans, grapes and cucumbers.

49 Hide the remote

Unplug your TV, hide the remote control and break your square-eyed habit. Cutting down on the amount of TV you watch will give your brain and your immune system a significant boost.

Research has shown that over-indulgence in TV viewing leads to an increased risk of obesity and heart disease from higher cholesterol, caused by lack of exercise. Other risks include poor concentration – as the brain cells governing attention span are impaired – and learning problems, as a result of poor intellectual stimulation.

It can work the other way too. Some types of TV programme – as well as video games – over-stimulate the senses and can upset sleep patterns. Meanwhile, the light from TV and computer screens can suppress the key hormone melatonin, raising the risk of cell DNA mutations that can cause cancer.

There's no need to cut out TV watching altogether; just get out of the habit of switching it on the minute you get home or whenever you are bored. Sit down with the viewing guide and pick out the programmes you want to watch that week. Watch only those programmes, and when they're over, turn the TV off and keep it off. If the programmes you watch regularly are cancelled, don't replace them with new ones. Instead, decrease the time you spend in front of the TV and do something active instead. Read a book, go for a walk, ride a bike or take part in some other kind of healthy physical activity for at least an hour before you turn on the tube.

And try getting rid of your remote. It's impressive how much less television you'll watch if you have to get up every time you want to change channels or adjust the volume. In addition, it eliminates all those wasted hours you spend channel-surfing.

50 Get out and mingle

Your immune system likes it when you spend time with your friends.

Studies suggest that having friends helps people live longer. Research in the *Journal of Epidemiology and Community Health* indicates that socialising with friends is beneficial. Not only can good friends encourage you to take care of your health but their presence can actually help you live longer, according to this research. Australian scientists have shown that having friends around in old age can increase life expectancy, and that friends may encourage people to look after their health, helping reduce feelings of depression and anxiety at difficult times.

There is a large amount of data showing the value of nurturing, social support and cama-raderie. In one such study, researchers exposed people to a cold virus and then monitored how many contacts those people had with friends, family, co-workers and members of church and community groups. The more social contacts people had – and the more diverse the contacts – the less likely they were to catch the cold.

Another 2005 study adds further weight to the theory that social support networks may strengthen the immune system. This study found that social isolation and loneliness can actually impair the immune system. Researchers at Carnegie Mellon University found that lonely and socially isolated first-year students mounted a weaker immune response to the flu jab than other students.

The same study also showed that it's not the number of friends you have that impacts on immunity the most, but the quality of those friendships. You can have very few friends but not feel lonely. Alternatively, you can have many friends yet still feel lonely. It seems that feelings of loneliness impair the immune system's response following a dose of influenza vaccine, while having fewer friends does not as clearly affect the immune system.

All this research contributes to a growing body of evidence that meaningful relationships and social support can enhance the functioning of the immune system. So whether you have one good friend or 50, spend more time with them.

51 Don't let smoke get in your eyes

If you smoke, it's best to quit – and if you don't smoke, avoid smoky areas.

Everyone is aware of the potential catastrophic impact on health of smoking. It is better not to start at all, but the sooner a smoker quits the better.

Because the damage caused by smoking is cumulative, the longer a person smokes the greater the risk of developing a smoking-related disease, such as lung cancer or heart disease. Quitting not only saves money, but also has added health benefits. Within one year of quitting, the risk of a heart attack falls to about half that of a smoker, and within ten years, the risk of lung cancer falls to about half that of a smoker. In Britain, about 120,000 people a year die from smoking-related illnesses – that's more than 300 every day.

Even if you don't smoke, the dangers of passive smoking or spending time in areas where people smoke, are also well documented. Passive smokers also have an increased risk of lung cancer and poor health, so protect your immunity and stay away from smoky areas.

52 Hold hands

Hold hands with someone you love. Give or get a hug from a friend or treat yourself to a periodic massage. Your immune system will thank you for it. Touch is important for boosting immunity too. It seems that giving or getting hugs or other forms of touch can boost the activity of the natural killer cells that seek out and destroy cancer cells or cells that have been invaded by viruses. Your skin is the largest sense organ of your body and stimulation of the skin is an important part of healthy immune system function. Unfortunately, many of us are too busy for hugs and become touch starved.

Studies on animals that are touched or handled extensively in infancy also show more developed immune systems than animals who have received less touch. They suffer fewer infections and have a lower mortality rate than their lesser-touched counterparts.

Is it possible to enhance your own immunity with a periodic massage and the immunity of your partner, friends and/or children by touching or hugging them more? All the evidence suggests that touch does benefit our health.

53 Compose yourself

. . . .

If you haven't got one already, invest in an iPod
or similar MP3 player and download and listen to
your favourite music as much as you can.

Music's ability to alter mood and emotional
state has long been known anecdotally, and more
recently has been scientifically documented.
Likewise, it's well recognised that mental and
emotional states can alter autonomic nervous
system (ANS) activity and balance. The ANS,
in turn, can modulate virtually every aspect of
immune function. The interaction between
feeling states, immunity and autonomic
function has been highlighted by a number of
studies showing that negative emotions such as
anger and hostility stimulate sympathetic
activity, increase the cortisol/DHEA ratio and
suppress the immune system, while positive
emotional states such as appreciation, love and
laughter enhance parasympathetic activity,
increase physiological well-being, reduce the
cortisol/DHEA ratio and boost immunity.

In short, listening to music can boost your
immunity, but it has to be music you love.

Something that calms one person might stress another person out. Whether it's Beethoven or Britney, the secret lies in finding music that soothes your soul. Scientists at Montreal's McGill University found that listening to music that sent shivers down the spine or that gave people goose bumps stimulated the same feel-good parts of the brain that are activated by food and sex.

Music therapy is now an established health service similar to occupational therapy and physical therapy. It is used to treat patients with a variety of disorders, including cancer, immune deficiencies and chronic pain. The American Music Therapy Association adds that the benefits of music therapy also include anxiety and stress reduction, pain management and positive changes in mood. These can lead to improved respiration, lower blood pressure, lowered heart rate and a reduced need for pain medication.

But even better than listening to music is actually making or composing it yourself. Other research has found that people who took part in an amateur group-drumming session had greatly enhanced natural killer-cell activity afterwards.

54 Turn down the volume

Try to take control over the noise in your environment, even if it means wearing earplugs to block out the sound of your partner's snoring or asking the store or gym manager to turn down the music.

Noise pollution is a growing problem in our 24/7 wired world of technology, machinery and gadgets; but noise hurts more than your ears. Any unwanted and intrusive sound can trigger muscle tension, speed heartbeat, constrict blood vessels and cause digestive upsets – exactly the same responses your body has to being startled or stressed.

Chronic exposure to noise can lead to even longer-lasting changes in blood pressure, cholesterol levels and immune function. Researchers at Cornell University found that women who work in moderately noisy offices produce more of the stress hormone adrenaline and may be more vulnerable to heart disease than women who work in quiet offices. Even worse are unwelcome sounds you perceive as uncontrollable, such as car or house alarms, barking dogs, noisy neighbours, snoring partners and mobile phones.

You can keep noise to a minimum by wearing earplugs when appropriate, using a humidifier at night to block out traffic sounds or sitting in designated mobile phone-free areas on public transport. Hanging wall coverings, carpets or paintings on your wall to break up flat surfaces that reflect sound will also help. And if you can, try to designate a quiet place or time in your house – a room or time of day where or when you can relax without unwanted background noise. If your partner snores and you find it impossible to get an immune-boosting good night's sleep, consider using earplugs or sleeping apart. You may also want to ask your partner to discuss with their doctor the wide range of snoring remedies available.

55 Say grace

Whether you are religious or not, taking a moment to give thanks or say grace before meals can do your immune system a great deal of good.

In recent years scientists have taken a look at the influence prayer has on our health and well-being, and some fascinating results have emerged. In one preliminary study, researchers wanted to investigate whether prayer had a beneficial impact on digestion, so they measured the after-meal comfort of those who said grace and those who didn't. Volunteers were asked to rate their level of comfort and satisfaction on a scale of one to ten, with one being low and ten being excellent. They were then asked to sit down and enjoy a meal and rate their level of satisfaction afterwards – the average rating was three. On another day, the same group of people were asked to say a silent prayer of thanks and the number rose to four. On yet another day, one member of the group was asked to say a prayer of thanks aloud and the average score increased again. On the following day, each group member was asked to say the prayer aloud in unison before the start of the meal and the number rose further. Finally, all the group members prayed aloud in unison and held hands at the same time and the number rose to an average of eight. This study was preliminary and it is hard to draw conclusions about whether or not prayer does boost digestion, but it does suggest that prayer can increase feelings of well-being and satisfaction.

This study also raises the fascinating question of whether or not praying for someone who is ill or praying for yourself to get better can boost your immunity. In one study of 393 coronary care patients, 192 received prayer from anonymous patients while the other 201 received no prayer. Patients had no idea they were being prayed for and at the end of the study the patients who were prayed for experienced fewer medical complications than those who were not prayed for.

Prayer is not a miracle cure and will not keep you or someone you care about from getting ill, but there is no doubt that prayer can give people a boost of strength, courage and motivation, and that this in turn can boost immunity.

56 Change your light bulbs

Switching from cool white fluorescent lights to full-spectrum lights could boost your immune function in a manner similar to the boost you get from exposure to natural sunlight.

German researcher Dr Fritz Hollwich discovered that when subjects sat under standard cool white fluorescent lights, levels of stress hormones rose considerably. High levels of stress hormones are known to have a depressing effect on immune function. By contrast, those sitting under full-spectrum lights experienced no such rise in stress hormones; inspired by Dr Hollwich's research, German hospitals no longer use cool white fluorescent bulbs.

Others studies have found that switching to full-spectrum lights significantly reduced the number of workplace absences due to illness. So if you aren't able to get enough natural daylight during the day (*see* page 115), invest in some full-spectrum light bulbs and use them at home and at work.

57 Get a new best friend

Owning a pet can have surprising immune-boosting benefits. For nearly 25 years, research has shown that living with pets provides certain health benefits. Pets have been shown to help lower blood pressure and lessen anxiety, but now research indicates that they may also be able to boost your immunity.

It was once thought that if your family had a pet, the children were more likely to become allergic to the pet. A growing number of studies, however, have suggested that children growing up in a home with pets – whether it's a cat or dog, or on a farm and exposed to large animals – will have a lower risk of allergies and asthma.

In addition to boosting immunity and easing stress, the simple act of taking care of a pet – whether you own a dog, cat, rabbit or goldfish – can add structure to your day and make you laugh. Unless you're someone who really dislikes animals, has a severe allergy or are absolutely too busy to care for one, getting a new best friend may be one of the best investments in your health that you ever make.

58 Zone out

However busy your day, find some time to unwind, zone out or simply relax, even if you are at work.

Studies have shown that people who have learned to relax seem to be healthier and more resistant to illness. Refuelling through relaxing can reduce the heart rate, lower blood pressure, increase blood flow to major muscles, reduce muscle tension, reduce headaches and back pain, improve concentration and reduce emotional responses such as anger and frustration. Small wonder hospitals and clinics all over the world are prescribing relaxation to patients with a variety of different conditions. But you don't need to be ill to engage in relaxation. When practised as part of a daily routine, relaxation can improve health at almost every level.

Relaxation should not be the last item on your to-do list. A daily relaxation can significantly reduce wear and tear on your body and mind. Everyone has different ways of winding down. Most often, relaxing involves a change of pace from the daily grind. Some people practise relaxation techniques such as deep breathing, meditation, visualisation or progressive muscle relaxation. Others like to read, write in a journal, take a walk with a friend, enjoy a massage or simply sit and daydream. It is crucial that the activity is made a regular part of your schedule. The goal is to refocus the mind and disregard extraneous thoughts and distractions, whether you are at home or at work, especially at work where long hours spent sitting at a desk can strain your body and mind.

Breathing in and out slowly and steadily for five minutes, stretching or taking yourself on a mini mental holiday – when you close your eyes and let your mind drift to a place where you feel relaxed and happy – are all proven ways to help you relax and unwind, anytime, anywhere. If you use these relaxation techniques daily, as well as at times when you feel stressed or tired, you will not only have a greater sense of well-being but your immune system will work more effectively.

59 Put your mind over matter

Boosting your immune system may be as simple as closing your eyes and putting your mind over matter.

Research suggests that meditation can help produce antibodies against illness and also lift mood. More studies are needed in this area, but for now the benefits of meditation on your immune system should not be underestimated.

The method of meditation you choose is not as important as achieving the desired result that promotes inner peace and relaxation – a quiet mind. There are many different types of meditation and you may decide to learn a specific technique, but whatever you settle on, make sure you enjoy it and it feels right. If you're not very familiar with meditation, here are a few techniques:

General meditation: Find a quiet place and time when you won't be disturbed, close your eyes and clear your mind of any thoughts. Sit like this, attempting to eliminate all thoughts and experience total peace for whatever period of time feels comfortable. Beginners often find it difficult to meditate for more than five or ten minutes. If you find yourself in such a situation, don't despair. You will find yourself able to sit for longer and longer intervals as time progresses. If you have never meditated before, consider aiming to spend five minutes meditating.

When you feel comfortable with this, try to increase the time to ten minutes. When you feel comfortable with that, try to move to 15 minutes, and continue like this until you find a length of time that suits you.

Focused breathing: This is another very popular yet tremendously simple meditation. As in general meditation, find a quiet time and place where you won't be disturbed, close your eyes and clear your mind of any thoughts. From there, focus on your breathing. Focus on the in-breath and on the out-breath. This is also commonly known as 'conscious breathing', because in contrast to our normal breathing which we do not focus on or attempt to control, focused breathing is consciously monitored and controlled. You simply 'watch' yourself breathe, so to speak, and attempt to bring your breaths to a slow, rhythmic pace (whatever pace feels comfortable to you).

By focusing on your breath, you draw your attention to that, and eliminate random and unsettling thoughts, thereby creating a feeling of inner peace. To help focus on the breath, people will often draw their attention to the air entering the nostrils, and the air leaving the mouth. You may also wish to draw your attention to the rising and falling of your chest. Use whatever method you feel comfortable with. As for controlling the pace of your breath, some people count a certain number of seconds between each breath and attempt to maintain this slow, rhythmic, controlled pace. Others prefer not to count. Still others use different techniques. Use whatever feels comfortable for you.

60 Visit your dentist

Studies have shown that there may be a link between poor dental health and an increased risk of heart disease, so take care of your teeth and visit your dentist regularly.

The explanation for the link between heart disease and gum disease may be that the bacteria that cause gum disease migrate throughout the body via the bloodstream and stimulate the immune system, causing inflammation that leads to the clogging of your arteries. Whatever the reason, the research underlines the importance of brushing and flossing twice a day and having a dental check-up every six to twelve months.

At your next dental appointment you may also want to ask your dentist to make sure you haven't got any mercury fillings. Mercury is known to damage the brain and nervous system, the thyroid, pituitary and adrenal glands, the heart and lungs, as well as hormone production. Research also appears to show that mercury released from dental fillings when you chew can bring about changes in bacteria that cause them to be resistant to antibiotics, thereby lowering the efficiency of your immune system.

100 Immune System Boosters

61 One-minute stress busters

Stress jacks up your body's production of cortisol and adrenaline, stress hormones that lower immune response. No wonder you're more likely to come down with a cold or the flu when faced with stressful situations such as final exams or relationship problems. Stress-induced anxiety can also inhibit natural killer-cell activity. Building some relaxation into your day, eating healthily, exercising regularly and getting a full night's sleep can help block the release of stress hormones and increase immune function in the long term, as can well-known relaxation techniques such as yoga, meditation and prayer.

For short-term stress relief when you're feeling tense, the following easy relaxation techniques will help bring you instant calm:

Don't take a deep breath: Ignore any advice to calm down and take a deep breath. It can make things worse. What you need to be aiming for are slow, steady breaths, not big, deep ones.

Breathe between sentences: Speaking quickly and taking gasps of air between long sentences can make your breathing too rapid and rack up stress and tension. Slow down your speech and remember to take a small breath after every sentence.

Breathe through your nose: When you feel you're losing control of your breathing and your peace of mind, breathing through your nose rather than your mouth makes the air the right temperature and humidity to encourage relaxation.

Work on your posture: Maintaining good posture is essential to relaxed breathing. If you're hunched or slouched there isn't enough room for your diaphragm to work effectively.

Shrug it off: Shrugging your shoulders helps release tension held in your neck and shoulders. Breathe deeply as you do the following exercise. Slowly and deliberately raise your shoulders as close to your ears as you can, and then push them backwards and down in a circular motion. Return to a relaxed position.

Try a few stress-busting scents: Certain essential oils have relaxing properties. Try sprinkling a few drops of relaxing herbal essential oil, such as lavender or sweet marjoram, on a tissue or handkerchief and sniff it as needed.

62 Shake off the talcum powder

Could your cosmetics, toiletries, make-up or skin-care products be making you sick?

The answer might be 'yes'. Scientists have shown that chemicals in cosmetics can pass through the skin and into the bloodstream and internal organs, so we should be more aware of what is being absorbed into our skin.

Talc particles have been linked to an increased risk of tumours in the lungs and breast. Your best bet is to stay away from talc and try other alternatives, such as mineral powders, cornstarch or rice powder for oil absorption.

Here are some more products to be wary of: coal tar, found in eye shadow, is also linked to cancer. Lipstick can contain high levels of artificial colourings made from coal tar derivatives, which can cause allergic reactions. Nitrosamine, a preservative, has been found in foundation creams, cured meats, pesticides, water, even air. Some epidemiological studies have associated increased incidence of human cancers with the presence of nitrosamine. Formaldehyde – the same stuff that preserves deceased bodies – is used in make-up, bubble bath, shampoos, conditioners, moisturisers and a whole lot more.

A few more to avoid are paraben preservatives and propylene glycol. Parabens were developed in the 1930s to stabilise creams and are now used in nearly all skin-care products. Researchers have recently found that there may be a connection between paraben preservatives and both breast cancer and male reproductive problems. Propylene glycol, which is used as a wetting agent, is an active ingredient in industrial antifreeze. It may cause kidney and liver abnormalities and even damage cell membranes. And finally, aluminium and other dangerous chemicals linked to an increased cancer risk have also been found in deodorants and antiperspirants.

Until more is known about their long-term health risks, it's best to play safe and buy natural toiletries and cosmetics as much as possible. If a product isn't natural, then it's important to read the label before purchasing. It's also a good idea to refresh your make-up every three to six months, as old make-up is a breeding ground for bacteria.

63 Battle a sick office

....

Your office or workplace could be making you sick, literally.

Most common ailments, such as flu, stem from an unhealthy workplace. Long hours hunched over a computer can cause eye and muscle strain, as well as bad posture. Bad posture can lead to muscular and even gastric ailments. These in turn can cause eye problems and conditions like carpal tunnel syndrome (the nerve on the wrist gets compressed due to handling the mouse, causing muscle weakness and pain).

The air you breathe can likewise be a major cause of concern. Lack of clean air can cause dehydration, fatigue, headaches and watery eyes. Air conditioners are a breeding ground for diseases such as Legionnaires' disease and asthma. Extremes in temperatures at your office can also cause the weakening of your immune system.

Here are a few signs that you just might be falling ill as a result of your office or workplace environment:

- Nagging eye problems, even ones as simple as eye irritation that does not go away even after rinsing with cool water.
- Recurrent health problems such as flu, cough and cold, body aches and headaches. These should be checked out in order to rule out more serious problems.
- Body rashes. These could indicate some chemical irritant around your workstation or in the air.
- Dust on your desk or in your workplace.

Some simple steps you can take:
- Confirm with office maintenance that they are cleaning the ventilator shafts regularly.
- Maintain a comfortable temperature in the office throughout the day.
- Equipment such as photocopiers and vending machines should be kept in a separate room.
- If your office has a carpet, make sure it is vacuumed at least once a week.
- Put an antiglare screen on your computer or wear computer glasses.

64 Start with your desk

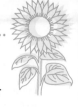

The more time you spend at your desk, the more germs accumulate there. Your desk may have about 400 times more bacteria than your office toilet seat.

Contrary to popular belief, it's virtually impossible to catch diseases from your toilet seat. Whatever micro-organisms there are on the seat's surface very rarely infect or contaminate the skin on your thighs and buttocks.

Most people believe that public areas like restrooms are havens for a whole panoply of germs. But the ugly truth is that there are more germs residing on your own office or study desk than on a public restroom toilet seat. Restrooms usually get cleaned and disinfected at regular and frequent intervals. But most people don't disinfect the things they use every day in their workplaces – including the desk, the phone and the computer keyboard and mouse.

Of all your office equipment and furniture, your phone has the most bacteria per square centimetre. Use a disinfectant wipe to clean it regularly. Your desktop, keyboard and then your computer mouse should be next in your anti-germ warpath. The average desk surface is home to thousands of bacteria just waiting to make you sick, so it might be wise to disinfect it now and again, especially if you eat lunch at your desk. Even your office supplies, such as your pen, can be a hidden harbour for germs. It's been estimated that accountants' and bankers' pens carry about 2,400 germs per 6.5 square cm (1 square in). Fax, photocopier and printer buttons, as well as the ground floor lift button, also have a lot of germs because so many people touch them.

This doesn't mean you should become paranoid and wear protective gloves to work. It just means that you should apply the same standards of cleanliness at work in your office as you would at home.

65 Toss out dead leaves

It's not just the germs on your desk, but also allergens on house plants that can be harmful to your health. So don't over-water your plants and keep their leaves well trimmed.

Dead leaves are a ripe food source for mould that can trigger allergic reactions. If you have clay pots, dust can collect on the outside of them, which will cause mould-eating mites to invade. House mould allergies have been linked to a number of health concerns, including asthma, fatigue and chronic coughing.

Bathroom condensation, shower curtains, leaky areas of the roof, plumbing leaks and water seepage in the basement can all attract mould.

The best way to avoid moulds is to take pre-emptive action. Take care of your plants by regularly trimming and removing dead leaves, keep plumbing in good repair, and try to maintain an indoor humidity of between 30–40 per cent. Remove items that have been contaminated by moulds, including carpet, if necessary.

66 Use your landline

Use your mobile phone for short calls only; save the long conversations for your landline.

There is considerable debate about whether electromagnetic fields have an adverse effect on immune function. But a growing number of researchers are beginning to uncover a link between lowered immunity and certain electromagnetic frequencies (EMF) emitted from mobiles, computers and other electrical devices such as TVs and microwaves.

Although the risks of electrical sensitivity are open to debate, until more is known protect your health by following common-sense safety guidelines. Mobile phones appear to be the worst culprits, so if you want to chat for a couple of hours use your landline instead of your mobile, and use other electrical appliances with care. Take regular breaks every half an hour or so when you work on your computer, switch the TV off when you have watched a specific programme, use batteries in your alarm clock, and cook and prepare healthy food instead of blasting all the goodness out of it in a microwave.

67 Now wash your hands

Hand washing is a simple habit – one that requires minimal training and no special equipment. Yet without doubt it's one of the best ways to avoid getting sick.

Regular and consistent hand washing is crucial for good health because throughout the day you accumulate germs on your hands from a wide variety of sources, such as direct contact with people, contaminated surfaces, foods, even animals and animal waste. If you don't wash your hands frequently enough, you can infect yourself with these germs by touching your eyes, nose or mouth. You can also spread these germs to others by touching them or by touching surfaces that they also touch, such as doorknobs, towels and taps.

Infectious diseases commonly spread through hand-to-hand contact include the common cold, flu and several gastrointestinal disorders, such as infectious diarrhoea. Inadequate hand hygiene also contributes to food-related illnesses, such as salmonella and *E. coli* infection.

Many of us simply put our hands under running water thinking that this will be sufficient, but it is important to use soap (you don't need antibacterial soap, regular soap is fine) and to wash thoroughly to make sure your hands are as germ-free as possible. The combination of scrubbing your hands with soap and rinsing them with water loosens and removes bacteria from your hands. Remember those scenes from TV hospital dramas? Doctors always scrub their hands meticulously, because they understand the health risks of dirty hands.

How to wash your hands properly

- Wet your hands with warm, running water and apply liquid or clean bar soap. Lather well. Rub your hands vigorously together for at least 15 seconds.
- Scrub all surfaces, including the backs of your hands, wrists, between your fingers and under your fingernails.
- Rinse well for about 20 seconds.
- Dry your hands with a clean or disposable towel.
- Use a towel or tissue to turn off the tap.

68 Wash your hands, PLEASE!

Although it's impossible to keep your bare hands completely germ-free, there are times when it's critical to wash your hands to limit the transfer of bacteria, viruses and other microbes. Always wash your hands – and if it isn't possible to wash your hands, avoid touching your face:

- After using the toilet.
- After changing a nappy.
- After touching animals or animal waste.
- Before and after preparing food, especially raw meat, poultry or fish.
- Before eating.
- After blowing your nose, or coughing and sneezing into your hands.
- Before and after touching a sick person.
- After handling rubbish.
- After using a cashpoint machine.
- Before inserting or removing contact lenses.
- After using taps and door handles that have been touched by others.
- After using handrails on escalators and lifts or buttons on lifts.
- After using the petrol pump.

69 A lot of flannel

Don't let your face flannel stay in a damp heap after you've used it. Put it in the laundry basket or hang it up to dry.

The warm and damp atmosphere of a bathroom encourages the growth of bacteria and germs that can make you ill. Soapy water loaded with bodily bacteria collects in thin layers on the surfaces of the shower, the bath and the shower curtain. If the curtain is made of fabric then it may be machine-washable at a low temperature. Face flannels remain popular, but their almost constant humidity makes them an ideal breeding ground for germs. As a result, they should be changed regularly and be made from thin material that dries quickly.

To keep your bathroom as hygienic and germ-free as possible:

- Clean and disinfect baths, sinks and toilets regularly.
- Clean your shower curtain regularly.
- Hang towels and face flannels up to dry after use.
- Give each family member their own towel.
- Air the room regularly to help disperse steam.

70 Get down and dirty

Spend more time in your garden or playing in the park as it could boost both your mood and your immunity.

The common belief that has driven medicine, as well as public perception and hygiene practices, is that when we get sick it is because of something we ate, inhaled or were exposed to in some way. The hygiene hypothesis, however, points in a different direction, proposing that with regard to many diseases it is precisely a lack of exposure to the bad guys that causes harm.

The argument is – and we don't yet have proof of it – that the immune system needs some kind of hardening, some kind of resistance, to function optimally. This doesn't mean you should abandon the health-boosting practice of hand washing – it just means that getting dirty isn't something you should always try to avoid (as long as you wash your hands afterwards).

While the evidence is by no means clear-cut, some studies show that children who lived on farms when they were very young have a reduced incidence of asthma, which has led several researchers to conclude that organisms in cattle dust and manure may be the stimuli that their immune systems needed to fight off asthma. The very latest research has shown that getting dirty in the garden can not only make your garden happy, it can boost your immunity and make you happy too. Exposure to dirt may be a way to lift mood as well as boost the immune system. Lung cancer patients treated with friendly bacteria normally found in the soil have anecdotally reported improvements in their quality of life.

Now that makes gardening the ultimate positive immune-boosting pastime. If you don't have a garden, find other ways to get down and dirty more often, such as walking around barefoot, digging in the dirt or playing football with your kids.

71 Change your tea towels

Dirty, damp cloths are the perfect breeding ground for bacteria, so it's very important to change tea towels frequently, and also to wash kitchen cloths and sponges regularly and leave them to dry before re-using them.

Although the average kitchen sink harbours up to 100,000 times more germs than a bathroom or toilet, most people consider the bathroom and toilet to be the most contaminated part of the house. Follow the guidelines below to keep your kitchen as healthy and germ-free as possible:

- Wash hands thoroughly before touching food. This is even more important after having touched a pet or used the toilet. Use waterproof plasters to cover cuts.
- Make sure that the sink and surrounding areas are cleaned regularly.
- Keep the fridge at a constant temperature of between 0–4°C (32–39°F and clean it, as well as cupboards, as often as possible. Put raw meat in a dish or on a plate.

- Always check that cleaned surfaces such as worktops and fridges are thoroughly dry before putting food down.
- Always wash any kitchen surface that has had uncooked meat on it to protect yourself against the risk of food poisoning. You should also separate any raw meat from cooked foods and don't use chopping boards, knives or utensils that have been used on uncooked meat on any other foods until they have been properly disinfected.
- Always wash fresh fruits and vegetables thoroughly before using.
- Wash and disinfect the bin and the area around it (in case of spatters). Bins contain high concentrations of bacteria, so it is important to empty them every day and to wash them regularly.
- Towels, cloths and sponges used in the kitchen should be changed daily and always washed carefully, not when they look dirty or when you remember to do it.

72 Buy a new toothbrush

Change your toothbrush every six weeks and,
if you get ill, throw your toothbrush away.

Some dentists recommend that when you get
ill you should throw out your toothbrush right
away. This is because although you can't catch
the same cold or flu virus twice, the virus can
hop to another toothbrush and make another
family member sick. Because toothbrushes are
relatively warm and moist, viruses like them and
can live on the bristles for as long as they remain
wet. If you live alone, chuck the toothbrush
when your symptoms go away. And if it's a
bacterial infection, such as strep throat, you may
re-infect yourself with the same germ that made
you ill in the first place. In that case, throwing
out your toothbrush protects both you and the
rest of your family.

Another precaution: don't store toothbrushes
too close to the toilet. Even toilet bowls that
appear clean can be filled with germs; every time
you flush the toilet, thousands of bacteria and
virus particles are catapulted into the air, floating
at least 1.5 m (5 ft) up and out.

73 Wipe the table

Table surfaces are often covered with germs, so wiping a table before you eat makes sense.

But how you wipe the table is as important as whether or not you do so. The best method for germ-proofing a table surface is to wipe it down with a household disinfectant, using a disposable paper towel; you'll throw away the germs when you jettison the towel. Avoid using a sponge or washcloth that you've used to clean other areas of the kitchen. For instance, if you use a sponge that's been used to clean a surface where you've cut meat, you could actually spread more bacteria around. The germs from the raw meat can remain on the sponge, and then spread to anything that sponge touches. Doctors call this 'cross-contamination'.

So to avoid the health risks of cross-food contamination always sterilise and launder your washcloths, sponges and brushes. Change your tea towels every day. You should also use one specific cutting board for meats, another for vegetables and another for bread and other kinds of chopping.

74 Play musical chairs

If you find yourself sitting next to someone
who is ill, get up and move; try to open a window
and if that isn't possible, keep your nostrils and
lips moist.

Every time a sick person coughs, sneezes or
simply breathes, tiny germ-laden droplets are
expelled into the air. One cough can spread
10,000 infectious viruses over a distance of
6 m (20 ft). Inhale these germs and you run the
risk of getting sick too. Whether you do get sick
depends on many factors, including the
hardiness of your immune system. You can
help your immune system do the best possible
job by eating properly, and by getting enough
rest and exercise. But there are some other
factors. You are less likely to pick up an illness,
for instance, if you aren't sitting too close to
others and are travelling in a well-ventilated
vehicle. Air generally circulates on trains and
buses, where it enters through the windows
and doors. (In fact, it's a good idea to open the
window a crack if you find yourself sitting
next to someone with the sniffles.)

Airplanes, however, can be problematic. Because airplane doors and windows are kept securely shut, it's up to the plane's ventilation system to keep air fresh – and it doesn't always do a great job of it. That means you can be exposed to the same germs more than once. So if someone in seat 7C has a cold, you're at risk of catching it – even if you're in 43B.

Another problem on airplanes is that the humidity level is low, resulting in dry throat, lips and nasal passages. One way viruses enter the body is through cracks in the dry mucous membranes, so if you keep those areas moist, your protection is greatly enhanced. A virus may land on the surface of the mucous membrane, but it will not infect you if that area is kept moist.

For added protection against an airplane's dry air, carry a bottle of over-the-counter saline spray on the trip. Squirt the spray into your nostrils throughout the flight whenever you begin to feel dry. Apply lip balm to keep your lips moist.

75 Don't let the bed bugs bite

Air your bedroom and house as much as possible to reduce the risk of allergic reactions to dust mites and bed bugs.

Dust mites are found in all homes, even very clean ones. They are microscopic organisms that thrive in warm and humid houses with lots of food – human skin. These mites prefer to live in beds and, because we spend about a third of the day in bed, we inhale large quantities of dust mite allergens. Reducing their number or containing their presence means that allergic reactions, such as coughing, sneezing or difficulties breathing, become less severe or non-existent. There are several ways of dealing with dust mites and bed bugs, and these methods are often best combined. Use bedding that can be washed often, cotton sheets, washable bottom sheets and synthetic blankets or duvets. Don't use woollen blankets or quilts.

- Wash bedding at high temperatures – above 55 °C (130 °F).
- Air your bed regularly and if you can, leave bedding, duvets, pillows and mattress covers

hanging outside for an hour every day or as often as practical.

- Buy a new mattress if your current one is over five years old.
- Dust mites hate dry and cold air, so try to air your bedroom and house every day, and don't use an air humidifier, which will only make matters worse. If the lower edge of the window is moist when you wake up in the morning, there is too much humidity in the air.
- Don't allow smoking in the house.
- Replace fitted carpets with wooden flooring or reduce areas of carpets in your home.
- Buy rugs that you can wash frequently.

76 Leave your face alone

If you are the kind of person who touches their face, rubs their eyes a lot or chews their nails, break the habit or at least wash your hands before you do so.

Germs that make you ill can't be absorbed through healthy skin, which is as protective as a latex glove. The danger comes when the hand that has touched the infected phone, cashpoint machine, door handle, petrol pump or out-stretched hand then touches mouth, nose or eyes, areas through which germs can and do enter the body.

Avoid shaking hands with someone who is coughing and sneezing. If you can't, wash them as soon as you can. This is the single most important means of preventing cold virus infections.

To break the habit of nail biting or nose rubbing you need to find a habit to take its place. Whenever you have the urge to bite, rub or scratch, then do your new habit instead – try drumming your fingers or just staring at your hands. Just make sure it's not a bad habit.

77 Let the dust settle

Every now and again give yourself a week off the housework.

Getting obsessive about cleanliness and sterilisation will not guarantee that you won't get ill; in fact, if the hygiene hypothesis is to be believed (*see* page 156) it may actually increase your chances of poor health. There really is no need to keep every speck of dust at bay. In fact, we need bacteria; they are essential for boosting our immune system. As with so many other important things in life, once again a balanced approach seems to be the answer. As long as you wash your hands at appropriate times, don't allow dust and dirt to build up too much, and keep your living and working environment as clean as you can without becoming obsessive about it, you'll be getting the balance about right.

While no health expert would recommend wallowing in dust and dirt, at the other extreme, it's positively unhealthy to worry too much about cleaning. Life, after all, is for living, not for cleaning. So put the duster and vacuum cleaner away, and have some fun instead.

Boosting immunity with supplements

Warning: Consult your doctor or pharmacist before taking any nutritional supplements, as large doses can be toxic. You should also ask your doctor if it is safe for you to take supplements if you are on medication, pregnant (or hoping to be), or have a pre-existing medical condition.

Likewise, it is essential to talk with your doctor or pharmacist before using herbal supplement. Just because herbal remedies are considered natural doesn't mean they're harmless. Herbal supplements can cause severe reactions with any prescription and over-the-counter medications you're taking, and can complicate other health conditions you may have. So be sure to tell your doctor or pharmacist about any herbal remedies you use.

78 Take out a nutritional insurance policy

The first step to boosting your immunity through nutrition is to eat a nutrient-rich diet. A healthy diet is one of the best things you can do for immunity and in an ideal world we would be able to get all our nutrients from the food we eat. However, this isn't an ideal world; we live in a time when our food is often nutrient-depleted due to modern farming techniques and the methods used in the processing of food.

Studies have shown those who take a daily multivitamin and mineral supplement have fewer infections than those who do not. It might, therefore, be a good idea to start your day by taking an all-round, high-quality supplement with a large glass of filtered water. A multi-vitamin should never be a substitute for a healthy diet, however, as the healthiest way to get your nutrients is through your food. Think of your daily multivitamin and mineral supplement as your insurance policy, or if you prefer, the icing on your cake.

If you're susceptible to colds or have a cold, supplement your diet with additional vitamin C.

Vitamin C is known to be a potent immune-stimulating nutrient. It increases the production of infection-fighting white blood cells and antibodies, and increases levels of interferon – the antibody that coats cell surfaces – preventing the entry of viruses. It also reduces the risk of cardiovascular disease by raising levels of HDL (good) cholesterol while lowering blood pressure and interfering with the process by which fat is converted to plaque in the arteries. People whose diets are high in vitamin C have lower rates of colon, prostate and breast cancer than those with a low intake. As a bonus, vitamin C supplementation may also reduce the severity of the common cold.

You don't have to take in massive amounts of vitamin C to boost your immune system. Opinions differ, but around 1,000 mg a day seems to be a generally agreed-upon amount and one that can be obtained by eating at least six servings of fruits and vegetables a day. If you take vitamin C supplements, it's best to space them throughout the day rather than take one large dose, most of which may end up being excreted in your urine.

Just as important to your immune system is vitamin E, which stimulates the production of natural killer cells, those that seek out and destroy germs and cancer cells. Vitamin E enhances the production of B cells, the immune cells that produce bacteria-destroying anti-bodies. Vitamin E supplementation may also reverse some of the decline in immune response commonly seen in ageing.

In addition, vitamin E can lower the risk of cardiovascular disease. In a Harvard School of Public Health study of 87,000 nurses, vitamin E supplementation was shown to cut the risk of heart attacks by 50 per cent. It's not difficult to obtain 30–60 mg of vitamin E daily from a diet rich in seeds, vegetable oils and grains, but it's difficult for most people to consume more than 60 mg a day consistently through diet alone. Supplements may be necessary to get enough vitamin E to boost your immune system.

80 Get a complex

If you're feeling stressed, run down or think you might be catching a cold, a vitamin B complex supplement may be the tonic your immune system needs.

Not a single substance but a group of water-soluble vitamins that combine with other nutrients to participate in a variety of oxidative enzyme systems, the B vitamins play a crucial part in maintaining the health of your immune system. The B vitamins work together and are needed for antibody production, ensuring that the immune army of white cells does their job properly. Vitamin B complex also helps to maintain a healthy digestive system, and is needed for healthy hair, skin and nails. The health of your mouth can also suffer if your diet is low in the vitamin B complex; mouth ulcers, for example, have been related to vitamin B deficiencies.

Wholegrains and cereals, liver, meat, poultry, fish, milk, eggs, leafy green vegetables, brewer's yeast, yeast extract and fortified breakfast cereals are good sources of vitamin B. If your diet isn't too good, if you are a vegetarian or are simply feeling run down, vitamin B complex supplements can make up for any deficiencies you may have in your diet. Some vitamin B complexes may not contain all eight of the essential B vitamins (thiamin B1, riboflavin B2, niacin B3, pantothenic acid B5, pyridoxine B6, cyanocobalamin B12, biotin and folic acid), so do count them on the label!

If you're taking a multivitamin and mineral supplement, you may already be getting your daily recommended intake of vitamin B complex, but check the label or talk to your pharmacist to make sure.

Warning: Be aware that high levels of vitamin B complex can be toxic so always follow the dosage instructions on the label, and don't exceed the suggested amount.

81 Don't give up on echinacea

The most popular immune-boosting herb today is echinacea. A flurry of recent studies has suggested that echinacea doesn't prevent the common cold; earlier research, however, shows that when taken at the first sign of a cold, it can still reduce cold symptoms and duration.

Although this herb is native to North America, most of the research studies have been carried out in Germany. Echinacea has been shown to be an effective antiviral agent against colds and flu, and the majority of effects appear to be due to the binding of echinacea polysaccharides to carbohydrate receptors on the cell surface of macrophages and T cells. Despite all this research, there has been continued doubt about the effectiveness of echinacea, but at long last it seems that scientists are finally coming round to the conclusion that it definitely does work.

In June 2007, an American team reviewed 14 studies using echinacea for prevention or treatment of colds, and published their results in the medical journal the *Lancet*. They found that the herb cut the chances of catching a cold by an average of 58 per cent, while reducing the duration of a cold by 1.4 days.

The antiviral action of echinacea not only helps you fight off a cold or combat flu, but it can also help build your immune system response, making it less likely that you will catch the next bug doing the rounds. Because the herb is also antibacterial and anti-inflammatory, it can deal with any bacterial infections or inflammations that may complicate the picture.

Given the amount of evidence to suggest echinacea's immune-boosting potential, taking echinacea at the first sign of a cold may be one of the best ways to build your defences. Echinacea is best taken as capsules of the powdered herb or as drops of a concentrated extract. Don't, however, take echinacea for longer than eight weeks as after that, the herb may over-stimulate the immune system.

82 Sip a soothing cuppa

Trade at least one cup of coffee each day for an energising green tea or a sugary fizzy drink for a soothing chamomile tea. To derive the optimal amount of immune-boosting nutrients from your tea, let the bag steep for at least three minutes in hot water.

Chamomile, according to researchers from London's Imperial College, is the herbal tea that'll help kick your cold into touch. In their recent study, people who drank five cups of the brew a day for two weeks had increased blood levels of plant-based compounds called polyphenols, some of which have been associated with greater antibacterial activity. Levels remained high for two weeks after subjects stopped drinking the tea. Chamomile tea also raised levels of glycine, a mild nerve relaxant and sedative.

Green tea is a rich source of a family of antioxidants called 'catechins', and preliminary research has found that a specific catechin – epigallocatechin gallate (egcg) – may give the beverage antigen-fighting abilities. When researchers at the University of Sherbrooke in Canada added green tea to lab samples of the adenovirus (one of the many viruses that causes colds), they discovered that egcg inhibited the virus's ability to replicate. Similarly, researchers in South Korea found that egcg can also stop the influenza virus from replicating. Although these studies were conducted in petri dishes instead of human subjects, some researchers believe you can reasonably bank on green tea's benefits – especially when it's consumed in place of fizzy sugary drinks with few nutritional benefits.

When you drink your tea, try to put your feet up for a few moments. Stress is a well-known inhibitor of the immune system and as more and more of us lead busy lives the humble tea break can be a real lifesaver.

83 Butter yourself up

Butterbur may sound like something that makes you sneeze, but the herbal supplement may actually help you fight allergies.

Butterbur is a shrub-like plant of the genus *Petasites* found in northern Asia, Europe and parts of North America and is currently being studied as a natural allergy treatment. Although the exact means by which butterbur works remains unknown, it is thought to have an effect similar to allergy medications, which block the action of histamine (inflammatory chemicals involved in allergic reactions).

In a study of 186 people with hay fever, participants took either a higher dose of butterbur (one tablet three times a day), a lower dose (one tablet two times a day) or a placebo. After two weeks, both the higher and lower doses relieved allergy symptoms as compared with the placebo, but there were significantly greater benefits seen with the higher dose. Scottish researchers found that patients with grass and pollen allergies who took 50 mg of the plant extract twice daily had a 13 per cent better nasal airflow than those who took the placebo.

Another study published in the *British Medical Journal* reported that butterbur treated seasonal allergies nearly as well as prescription medications. It is effective against all symptoms of allergic rhinitis, including sneezing, itching and conjunctivitis, because it can block the action of leukotriene, a chemical that causes allergic reactions, while at the same time controlling white blood cells that accumulate when allergic reactions take place.

If you suffer from allergies, butterbur is safe to take for up to two weeks; studies have not been done to see if it is safe or effective in the long term, so don't take it for longer than two weeks. There are no drowsy effects with butterbur, and you can buy it in supplement form at most health food stores.

84 Go mushrooming

Certain kinds of mushrooms have been used for centuries in China and Japan to boost immunity. The most popular are shiitake, maitake and reishi.

In 1960, Dr Kenneth Cochran (an American herb researcher at the University of Michigan) carried out a series of studies on the properties of shiitake mushrooms. He discovered that shiitake has a strong antiviral compound called lentinan that stimulates the immune system. In follow-up research conducted in Japan, shiitake proved more effective than a powerful prescription drug in fighting viruses. It was also effective against many types of viral infections.

The maitake mushroom is gaining recognition as a powerful means of strengthening the body and enhancing the immune system. The polysaccharides found in maitake have exhibited the highest cell-protecting quality of any mushroom and are considered one of the most potent forms of immunological stimulation. Reishi mushrooms can also increase bodily resistance against cell mutation and enhance immune function.

85 Try a herbacure

Although echinacea and butterbur are among the most well-known medicinal herbs, they are not the only immune-boosting super herbs around. The following herbs are readily available from health food stores and chemists, and can all be used to help boost your immunity and build stamina. Why not give one a try?

Aloe vera: This wonderful herb contains a whole host of beneficial substances, including vitamins, minerals, amino acids, enzymes, essential fats and a most potent immune booster called acemannan that has been shown to support immune function by increasing the number and function of T cells.

Astragalus: A Chinese herbal remedy that comes from the root of a plant in the pea family, astragalus is used to combat colds, flu and other respiratory infections. It has excellent antiviral, as well as immune-enhancing properties, and is ideal for those who catch colds easily or suffer from lowered immunity.

Elderberry: Working as a natural diuretic, sambucol (or black elderberry extract) helps improve immune function and enhances overall energy and vitality. It appears to be particularly effective against the influenza virus. In a double-bind clinical trial, more than 90 per cent of the 15 patients taking elderberry extract showed a significant reduction in influenza symptoms after two days, and complete recovery after three days. However, in the control group it took six days before 90 per cent of patients showed an improvement. The group taking elderberry extract also had higher levels of influenza antibodies in their blood than the control group, indicating an enhanced immune response.

Garlic: Just eat it; don't spend money on a supplement! Garlic is a wonderful all-round, powerful addition to your diet. It has antiviral, antifungal and antibacterial properties, and is more potent if you can stomach it raw.

Liquorice: A tincture of liquorice root may be effective against Candida and several other types of bacteria. According to laboratory studies, a compound in liquorice impairs the ability of viruses – including herpes – to survive.

Peppermint: Taken as an infusion (either fresh or dried), peppermint is a powerful decongestant. Just holding your nose above a cup of warm peppermint tea and inhaling the steam will soon clear your sinuses. It's valuable when there are colds and flu about, and also helps to settle upset stomachs.

There are many other herbs and plant extracts that may be able to boost immunity and some – such as bioflavonoids (found in citrus fruit), quercetin (found in cranberries) and grape extract – are sold separately as immune-boosting remedies. Others such as thyme, lemon, cinnamon, cardamom, turmeric, oregano, parsley, cloves and ginger can be used to spice up your cooking.

Essential oils not only ease stress but are also antiseptic and antiviral, so they can help soothe symptoms of a cold or flu by killing bacteria and soothing inflamed membranes. The combined antiviral and uplifting properties of essential oils can also help keep bugs at bay, while keeping you feeling refreshed at the same time.

Put essential oils into a vaporiser in places where viruses tend to lurk, such as on your desk at work or in your car. Alternatively, place a few drops of essential oil on a handkerchief to inhale whenever your immune system needs a pick-me-up.

Warning: Do not apply neat (undiluted) essential oils to the skin. They are potent substances and should always be diluted in a carrier oil such as olive, almond or grapeseed oil (5 drops of essential oil to 10 ml (1 tablespoon) of carrier oil).

Cinnamon: Great for boosting the immune system, it has been shown to support the pancreas and digestive system (in Chinese medicine, the pancreas/spleen relates to the immune system). Apply on the feet or inhale.

Lavender: One of the most widely used and effective of the essential oils, it is generally not used in the acute stages of bacterial infection, but can be used to boost immunity.

Lemon: Like cinnamon, lemon essential oil has positive effects on the immune system. Take a drop or two in every glass of water you drink throughout the day or take in capsule form. Lemon is photosensitive, so it should not be applied to skin.

Peppermint and eucalyptus: These oils are cool and soothing, and are both known to clear the respiratory system and ease breathing. They can be applied in diluted form directly to the neck, throat, chest and back to open the lungs, or can be inhaled to soothe the sinuses. Peppermint and eucalyptus are safe to apply on the skin in diluted form.

The same essential oils that you might use to treat a virus, cold or flu can also be used as prevention. If your workplace is full of sniffly people or half your child's classmates have been sick this week, now might be a good time to start using these oils. A drop of oregano oil on the bottom of your feet in the morning, lemon in your glass of water at lunch or lavender in your vaporiser can go a long way towards boosting your immune system and preventing you from catching the latest bug doing the rounds.

Essential oils contain hundreds of molecules that work together to kill bacteria and viruses and to support your body's health. Unlike drugs, viruses do not develop resistance to essential oils because each batch of oil is unique depending on a growing season's temperature range, time of harvest, etc. For this reason essential oils can be more effective at beating cold and flu than drugs.

87 Go hot and cold

Soak your feet in hot water for a few minutes
and then splash your feet with cold water to give
yourself a little immune-boosting hydrotherapy.

The therapy encompasses a variety of healing
treatments that involve water, including ice packs
and hot baths. Different water temperatures, often
alternated, are used to achieve certain effects.
For example, hot water dilates blood vessels,
increasing blood flow to the skin and muscles.
This improves circulation and stimulates the
immune system. Waste products are effectively
removed, while nutrients and oxygen are carried
around the body. Cold water, on the other hand,
stimulates the blood vessels near the skin's surface
to constrict, sending blood away from the skin
and towards the internal organs, improving their
functioning and reducing inflammation.

The idea that nature has healing properties is
an age-old concept, and water has always been
a part of nature's therapeutic toolkit. You are
employing the healing effects of hydrotherapy
when you put your sprained ankle in an icepack,
place a vaporiser in your coughing child's room
or use a damp washcloth to alleviate a fever.

88 DIY massage

Pamper yourself with a gentle massage. Your immune system will thank you for it.

Massage can relax the body, trigger the release of endorphins (the body's own painkillers) and induce feelings of comfort and well-being. It can also boost your immunity. Research among different groups of people in very different situations has shown that massage can increase the immune system's cytotoxic capacity (the activity level of the body's natural killer cells) and decrease the number of T cells. The result is an immune system that works better. Massage doesn't cure ailments, but it has been shown to help the body function better in fighting ailments.

A great way to boost your immunity is to book yourself in for a monthly massage, but if this isn't possible try the following DIY tension-busting massage techniques.

Feet: Using the palm of your hand, stroke the length of your foot from heel to toe, starting gently and applying more pressure on each stroke. Using your thumb, make deep circular movements on the soles of your feet, working across the entire sole before massaging each toe individually, placing it between finger and thumb, and rolling the toe between them.

Back: Lie on your back on the floor; clasp your knees up to your chest and gently rock from side to side, then forwards and backwards.

Shoulders: Place your palms on your temples and very slowly rotate your hands forwards, up and back several times. With your right hand on your left shoulder squeeze the hand together, making circular movements with the fingers. Repeat on the opposite side. This DIY massage is ideal for anyone who spends too long sitting in front of a computer.

Hands: It may seem surprising that people carry a lot of tension in their hands. But it's actually obvious when you think about how much hands are used. Most hand movements are holding actions, so it is relaxing to counter-act this by opening your palm and your fingers. As you do this with one hand, squeeze your hand and fingers all over with the other and make circular movements over the joints with your thumb.

89 Strike a pose

So what does yoga have to do with immunity? Quite a lot actually, as new research shows that yoga postures can help boost your immune system.

The 'warrior pose' is a powerful yoga pose that is thought to stimulate the lymph glands and white blood cell production, and boost immunity. To perform the warrior pose, position yourself on a non-slip surface (ideally a non-slip yoga mat). Stand upright, facing forwards and step the right foot 1 m (about 3 ft) to the right and place it at a 90° angle to the body. The left foot should remain facing forwards. Bend the right knee to almost a 45° angle keeping the upper torso facing forwards. Extend the right arm completely, making a fist with the thumb pointing up (as though you're holding an archery bow). Bring the left arm across the body to the right arm and pull back across the body and hold. Start by holding this pose for one minute and then perform the same series of moves on the left side.

90 Get in harmony for your health

Simply watching the graceful
movements of people practising
T'ai chi in the park is soothing,
but your immune system would benefit
more if you did some T'ai chi yourself!.

Originally developed in China as a form of
self-defence, T'ai chi is a graceful form of
exercise that has existed for some 2,000 years.
Practised regularly, T'ai chi can help reduce
stress. It is often described as 'meditation in
motion' because it promotes serenity through
gentle movements connecting the mind and
body. Recent research also suggests that T'ai chi
doesn't only improve flexibility and ease stress; it
can also strengthen the immune system.

To do T'ai chi, you perform a series of postures
or movements in a slow, graceful manner.
Anyone, regardless of age, can practise T'ai chi.
You don't need any special clothing or equipment and you can practise at home. To gain the
full benefits of the art, however, it is best to seek
guidance from a qualified T'ai chi instructor.

91 Pins and needles

Regular acupuncture sessions may boost your immunity and improve your resistance to infection.

Acupuncture is an age-old Chinese medical practice that involves the use of fine needles, placed at specific points along pathways of '*Qi*' (vital energy) in the body. Qi (also known as Chi) is part of a meridian system within the body and it is through this network that Qi flows or gets blocked as the case may be. This is based on the concept that blockage of Qi leads to poor health and lowered immunity; acupuncture is used to remove these blockages.

Acupuncture is currently being investigated as a means of stimulating immunity in people with AIDS and other immunosuppressive disorders. Although acupuncture is painless, if the idea of needles doesn't appeal then acupressure, a form of massage based on the same principle, may have similar immune-boosting benefits. Shiatsu, a Japanese form of bodywork which you might want to try, also uses pressure points to release blocked Qi.

Boost immunity with a fighting spirit

92 Look on the bright side

The immune system takes many of its cues from our thoughts and feelings, so try to keep your outlook upbeat.

Learning to be more positive is a skill anyone can master. You're in charge of everything that you think; once you start to recognise negative thought patterns, you can start challenging them and replacing them with more positive ones or, at the very least, more appropriate ones.

Negativity may seem like a personality trait that's difficult to change, but if wearing glasses with a rose-coloured tint can improve your immunity, why not try on a pair? Every time you hear yourself using negative words such as 'can't', 'won't', 'shouldn't', 'problem' or 'failure', replace them with positive words or phrases such as 'I can', 'I will', 'I'd like to', 'opportunity' and 'learning experience'.

93 Laugh out loud

Stop taking yourself so seriously. Find the humour in things and engage in activities that make you laugh, because laugher has been shown to increase your immune function and disease resistance.

Research shows that laughter may be beneficial to health. Laughing appears to stimulate digestion, ease stress, reduce muscle tension, lower blood pressure and boost blood flow; researchers have found that it may even reduce the risk of developing heart disease. One study found that people who responded to stress by seeing the humour or the bright side in the situation had higher blood levels of immunoglobulin A (a key antibody) than their gloomier counterparts.

While painful emotions such as anger and grief can impair health, laughter does the opposite. A real belly laugh increases infection-fighting antibodies and boosts natural killer-cell activity. Even anticipating or looking forward to a good time can enhance immunity, so the next time you plan ahead for the weekend, make sure there is plenty of time for fun.

Even if you did not grow up in a household where laughter was a common sound, you can learn to laugh at any stage of life. Begin by setting aside special times to seek out humour and laughter, as you do for exercise. Smiling more often is a great place to start. When you look at someone or see something even mildly pleasing, practise smiling. If nothing makes you chuckle think about all the good things in your life. If that still doesn't help spend time with people who naturally take life lightly, who routinely find ordinary events hysterical. Their points of view and their laughter are contagious.

Good sex is fun, feels great and is good for your health and immunity.

Sex reduces stress, leads to greater contentment and better sleep. Regular sex is regular exercise and has similar benefits, including improved cholesterol levels and increased circulation. Apart from giving you a good work out, sex once or twice a week improves the immune system as well. Researchers have found higher levels of immunoglobulin A in individuals who have regular sex. Immunoglobulin A is a type of antibody that helps to protect us from infections. It is normally found in high levels in the mucous membranes of the digestive and respiratory tracts.

Aches and pains? Studies have shown that sex reduces headaches and joint pain. In medical terms immediately before orgasm, levels of the hormone oxytocin surge to five times their normal level. This in turn releases endorphins, which alleviate both physical and emotional pain. So next time a headache threatens, reach for your partner instead of a pill.

95 Talk to your white blood cells

For a few moments each day imagine or visualise yourself positively glowing with health. Visualisation is the technique of using your imagination to create what you want in life. It is based on the principle that the mind and the body are intimately connected.

Visualisation is at the centre of relaxation techniques designed to release stress-busting brain chemicals that act as your body's natural brain tranquillisers, lowering blood pressure, heart rate and anxiety levels. By and large, researchers find that these techniques work. Several studies suggest that visualisation can also boost your immunity. Researchers at Ohio State University found that people with cancer who used visualisation while receiving chemotherapy felt more relaxed, better prepared for their treatment and more positive about their care than those who didn't use the technique. Danish researchers also found increased natural killer-cell activity among ten college students who imagined that their immune systems were becoming very effective. Natural killer cells are an important part of the immune system because they can recognise and destroy virus-infected cells, tumour cells and other invaders.

In another small-scale study, researchers at Pennsylvania State University and Case Western Reserve University School of Medicine found that seven people who suffered from recurrent canker sores in their mouths significantly reduced the frequency of their outbreaks after they began visualising that the sores were bathed in a soothing coating of white blood cells. Other studies have shown that visualisation can lower blood pressure, slow heart rate and help treat insomnia, obesity, anxiety, stress and phobias.

Visualisation, a form of self-hypnosis, is a technique anyone can use to boost their health and immunity. First quieten yourself by taking a few slow and steady breaths. Close your eyes and visualise yourself inhaling golden or white light (or energy), and exhaling grey, stale and old light. The golden or white light represents new, fresh, rejuvenating health and energy, while the grey light represents any stress, unhappiness or toxins that damage your health. If you have a specific ailment from which you're trying to relieve yourself, visualise the same white or golden light surrounding the area of your body that's in need of healing. Focus on the white or golden light healing and energising that area of your body. Continue focusing this healing light on the afflicted area of your body for whatever period of time feels comfortable to you. Try to repeat this procedure daily (or multiple times daily if you feel compelled to do so).

Alternatively, you could actually imagine a battle between your white blood cells and the virus or bacteria, with your white blood cells emerging as the conquering heroes. As always, do what feels right for you.

96 Write in a journal

Before you go to bed at night write down a few thoughts about your day, how you are feeling, and your hopes and dreams for the following day.

Writing in a journal every day is an immune-boosting stress release for many people. It is stress relieving not just to get thoughts and feelings out on paper, but also to be able to see a pattern and meaning in your life. Research has shown that cancer patients who see a purpose or meaning to their lives or have a fighting spirit, seem to live longer than those who are despondent.

If writing isn't your thing, anything that gives you a fighting spirit or sense of meaning and purpose in life – such as prayer, actively campaigning for a charity or cause or regular volunteer work – can help boost your immunity.

It would seem fairly obvious that helping others will make you feel good, but what about actual health benefits? Studies have shown that volunteering can play a role in increasing your overall sense of well-being, alleviating chronic pain and even reducing depression.

97 Do a crossword

Brainy games, such as crosswords, Sudoku, bridge or chess, may give both your brain and your immune system a workout.

Research shows that certain kinds of thinking may be able to boost immunity. Dr Marian Diamond, a neuroscientist at the University of California, Berkeley, found that playing bridge stimulated people's immune systems. Her research is the first to show a connection between the immune system and the part of the brain that handles planning, memory, initiative, judgment and abstract thinking.

More research needs to be done, but it seems that any mental activity that gets you fully absorbed using one or more of these intellectual functions might benefit your immune system. And, of course, it's not just your immune system that benefits from crosswords and other games that challenge your brain. Research shows that people who do these kinds of brainy games on a regular basis keep their brains more agile and starve off memory-loss associated with age, particularly short-term memory.

Make sure you make enough quiet time for yourself.

A few minutes alone every day in total peace and quiet can centre you for the whole day. Not only is this time alone desirable, quite honestly, it is necessary for mental health and well-being. It allows you to take a mental deep breath, to step back from active engagement in the day and to reflect a little.

Studies show that our bodies respond to our emotions – if you're feeling harassed and anxious, it can manifest in a sore throat or a cold. So create a space within your living environment where you can find some peace and quiet to gather your thoughts.

If this isn't possible, create a space inside yourself for harmony, self-love and joy (giving thanks, prayer and blessing the abundance in your life and in the world around you all count). Use your quiet space or quiet time to pay attention to warning signs of an immune system in trouble, such as headaches, fatigue or a sore throat, so you can keep them from getting worse. Remember, your body will tell you if your immune system is in danger so you need to listen to it on a regular basis and be aware of any slight changes. The earlier you recognise the signs and symptoms of weakened immunity the faster you can take corrective action and the more likely you are to avoid getting ill.

Remember, when you're calm and happy and in touch with your physical and emotional needs, you're far less likely to get sick. But when you are stressed and overloaded you are far more likely to get sick. In the past decade there is more than enough evidence to suggest that stress has an impact on your health. In fact, researchers have even coined a name for this new field of study. They call it psychoneuro-immunology. Quite a mouthful but all it really means is that constant stress can compromise our immune system, rendering it less effective in warding off bacteria and viruses.

99 Surprise yourself

Do something today to surprise yourself. Dare to be different. See life from a new perspective.

People who cling to rigid points of view and ways of doing things tend to be more susceptible to stress than people who are more open-minded and flexible in their approach to life, and stress is bad news for your immune system. Research shows that negative thinking, rigid routines and rigid ways of thinking are associated with stress, and longer and more severe infections. In other words, rigidity or inflexibility in your beliefs may translate into a rigid and inflexible immune system.

So keep your immune system on its toes and your life spontaneous by constantly surprising it with new stimuli. Take a new route to work, eat food you don't normally eat, sit in a different chair at dinner, wear a colour you haven't worn before or change your hairstyle. It doesn't matter what it is; just make sure it's different enough to wake your mind up so you can see life from a different perspective.

100 Stop and smell the flowers

Stop feeling guilty about doing the things you love.

Numerous studies show that seeking out pleasure can have a beneficial and measurable physiological and psychological effect on the pleasure-seeking individuals. So, whether it's spending time with loved ones, having your hair done or going out to the movies, don't feel guilty about doing the things you love. Your immune system thrives on it.

Breaking away from what you feel you ought to be doing or what you feel is more productive time is very difficult. Crossing a lot of things off a 'to-do' list is a great feeling, but what separates those who live healthy and fulfilling lives from those who are less healthy and happy is that the really healthy and happy people know how to manage their time more productively. Oftentimes, increased productivity comes not from working more, but from balance and better time management.

PART THREE:

FIGHTING INFECTION

Working out your immune system

If you do go down with a cold or flu, don't feel disappointed with yourself; most adults get two to three colds a year, and even the fittest, healthiest and happiest person will succumb now and again. Indeed, according to recent research, the odd infection may actually be good for you because it gives your immune system a workout. To put it another way, just as muscles and brain cells need to be used if you want to stay fit and mentally agile, you need to get ill every once in a while to keep your immune system fighting fit.

Medication

When you are down with an infection you can experiment with complementary therapies (*see* 'Part Two: Boosting immunity with supplements'), or consult your doctor or pharmacist for over-the-counter medication. If your temperature rises above 39°C (102F) despite taking anti-inflammatory drugs such as ibuprofen, be sure to seek medical advice immediately. This, combined with chest pains and shortness of breath, could be a sign of pneumonia.

Some medications can boost your immunity by reducing your susceptibility to infectious agents. For example, taking anti-parasitic medication can protect you against malaria if you live in an area that is high risk. Antihistamines can block the action of histamine and reduce allergy symptoms. And your doctor may also prescribe antibiotics to reduce the severity of symptoms during a bout of illness. However, overuse of antibiotics isn't advised as this can result in more resistant, harder-to-treat strains of bacteria.

Antibiotics are both a blessing and a curse. They are strong medications that can stop life-threatening illnesses – such as meningitis and pneumonia – and save lives; but if they aren't used correctly, they can be damaging. Frequent and inappropriate use of antibiotics can result in strains of bacteria that require even stronger antibiotics for successful treatment.

When to use antibiotics

The correct use of antibiotics is the best way to ensure that antibiotics remain useful in treating infection. Antibiotics will not work for infections caused by viruses and are only effective against infections caused by bacteria. This is why they are not appropriate for colds, flu, sore throats and most coughs, as these tend to be caused by viruses. The best thing to do with a cold or flu is to let it run its course and, if your illness gets worse after two weeks, to consult your doctor.

You should consult your doctor if there's a problem with your lungs, as bacteria may be the cause and your doctor may prescribe an antibiotic. Strep throat is also caused by bacteria and needs a course of antibiotic treatment. Some, but not all, ear infections and sinus infections will need to be treated with anti-biotics, so once again consult your doctor.

If you're prescribed a course of antibiotics, listen to your doctor's advice carefully. To protect your future immunity, make sure you take the full course prescribed and never share other people's anti-biotics or use an unfinished course for another illness.

DIY home remedies for colds and flu

With no cure in sight for the common cold, current treatments can at best only bring relief to symptoms by shortening their duration. Your best bet is to take it easy and make yourself as comfortable as possible; if you do treat your symptoms, make sure to treat them gently.

Don't forget that the uncomfortable and unpleasant symptoms you experience when you get ill are often best treated mildly because they are an indication that your immune system is doing its job. For instance, a fever is your body's way of trying to kill viruses by producing an environment that's hotter than normal; one or two days of moderate fever may help you get well faster. Coughing and sneezing are other signs of natural healing, as they are your body's way of trying to clear your breathing passages of the thick mucus that carry germs to your lungs. Even a stuffy nose is best treated mildly, as it is your body's way of warming the infected area in your nose and throat so that germs can be carried out of your body sooner rather than later.

You could also try some of the following tried-and-tested home remedies:

Fight flu with elderberry

In the 18th century, Europeans drank hot wine made from the berries of the elderberry tree to ease cold and flu symptoms. Modern herbalists still recommend elderberry for viral infections, especially the flu.

Stay warm and rested

Staying warm and rested when you first come down with a cold or the flu helps your body direct all its energy towards winning the immune battle. Fighting infection is taxing for your body, so help it along by putting your feet up and wrapping up warm under a blanket.

Gargle

This can relieve a dry throat and bring temporary comfort and relief. Try a teaspoon of salt dissolved in warm water, four times daily. To reduce tickling in your throat, try an astringent gargle (such as tannin-rich tea) to tighten the membranes. Or use a thick, soothing gargle made with honey. Steep one tablespoon of raspberry leaves or lemon juice in two cups of hot water and mix with one teaspoon of honey. Let the mixture cool to room temperature before gargling.

Eat lightly

If you start to come down with a cold or the flu, eat lightly so that your body can focus on healing. For the first 24 hours, drink filtered water and consume broths and soups with lots of immune-boosting garlic, onions and spices (turmeric and cayenne pepper work particularly well). These will relieve congestion, promote good circulation and have a natural anti-inflammatory effect. Herbal teas (especially ginger, cinnamon and peppermint) and steamed vegetables are also good choices. It's important to eat lightly when you have a fever; the old saying 'starve a fever, feed a cold' is quite correct, because loss of appetite is your body's way of saying that you should eat less while it battles invaders. When you're feeling better you can move towards a more normal diet.

Drink hot liquids

Hot liquids can relieve nasal congestion, prevent dehydration and soothe the uncomfortably inflamed membranes that line your nose and throat. So drink lots of hot water with lemon during the day, especially if you have a fever.

Chicken soup

Good old-fashioned homemade chicken and vegetable soup can be a great comfort when suffering from a cold or flu. It's warming and full of vital nutrients to help you get over your illness. Your soup should contain plenty of vegetables that are high in immune-boosting beta carotene (such as carrots, sweet potatoes, turnip greens and spinach). Adding herbs and spices can help bring relief and loosen up mucus. A pinch of cayenne pepper in your soup can help you fight off some of the aches and pains, as well as helping to reduce the fever.

When you feel better try some homemade carrot soup (*see* page 67) to stop you getting ill again.

Take a steamy shower
Steam can help moisturise your nasal passages and relax you. If you're dizzy or shivery from the flu, run a steamy shower while you sit on a chair nearby and take a sponge bath.

Blow your nose a lot and do it in the right way
It's important to blow your nose regularly when you have a cold or flu, rather than sniffling mucus and germs back into your head and down into your lungs and the rest of your body. But when you blow hard, pressure can carry germ-carrying phlegm back into your ear passages, causing earache. The best way to blow your nose is to press your finger over one nostril while you blow gently to clear the other. Do not forget after you have blown your nose to wash your hands.

Warm saltwater for stuffy noses
Saltwater rinsing helps break nasal congestion, while also removing virus particles and bacteria from your nose. To give your nose a saltwater rinse:

Mix ¼ teaspoon salt and ¼ teaspoon baking soda in 225 ml (8 oz) warm water. Using a bulb syringe to squirt water into your nose, hold one nostril closed by applying light finger pressure while squirting the salt mixture into the other nostril. Let it drain. Repeat two or three times, and then treat the other nostril.

Salve your nose

A small dab of mentholated salve under your nose can open breathing passages and help restore the irritated skin at the base of the nose. Menthol, eucalyptus and camphor all have mild numbing ingredients that may help relieve the pain of a nose rubbed raw.

Savour a curry

We have seen that the first half of the saying 'starve a fever, feed a cold' is correct; so is the second half. When you have a cold, eating hot foods such as chilli peppers, hot mustard, radishes, peppers, onions and garlic (which contain substances called mucolytics, similar to over-the-counter expectorant cough syrups) help liquefy the thick mucus that accumulates in the sinuses and breathing passages.

Foot bath
Try 2 teaspoons of fresh ginger in a foot bath to draw blood away from the head to the feet, which helps to reduce the heat and congestion you may feel in the rest of your body when ill. Adding one teaspoon of dried mustard to a bowl of hot water can also have a warming effect.

Apply hot or cold packs around your congested sinuses
Choose a hot or cold pack and apply gently to your congested sinuses; either temperature works, so choose the one with which you feel most comfortable. You can buy reusable hot or cold packs at a chemist, or you can make your own easily. Take a damp washcloth and heat it for 55 seconds in a microwave (test the temperature first to make sure it's right for you). Alternatively, take a small bag of frozen peas to use as a cold pack.

Extra vitamin C

In addition to eating plenty of vitamin C-rich fruits and vegetables and taking your daily multivitamin and mineral supplement, you might want to take extra vitamin C during a bout of illness. Vitamin C is an incredible antiviral agent and research has shown that vitamin C supplements can ease symptoms of colds and flu. Viruses cannot survive in a bloodstream saturated with vitamin C, so mix 6 g of vitamin C powder in fruit juice diluted with water and drink throughout the day. If you think you're feeling better, wait a day before reducing your vitamin C supplement to 1 g three times a day. Once you have been well for a few days, go back to your normal immune-boosting eating and supplement programme (*see* pages 168–71).

Zinc lozenges

Zinc lozenges are often found in health stores marketed as natural cold remedies. A number of studies have found that zinc helped to reduce the duration of cold symptoms, especially if people started taking it within 24 hours after the appearance of cold symptoms. It was also found to reduce the severity of symptoms and their duration by three or four days. Zinc lozenges may work by blocking the replication of the cold virus (preventing it from spreading) or by impairing its ability to enter cells in the nose and throat. Unfortunately, these studies suffered from several flaws and better-quality studies are needed; at this stage, at least, long-term use of zinc lozenges is not recommended.

Take probiotic supplements

The purpose of antibiotic drugs is to destroy pathogenic bacteria, but in the process they also destroy beneficial bacteria. A single course of antibiotics can wipe out beneficial bacteria for several months and overuse over several years can actually make you more vulnerable to viruses and infection. Probiotics, on the other hand, are not a drug used to wipe out the enemy, but a specific strain of beneficial bacteria that can reinforce the body's natural defences. They can be used to restore health in the digestive tract – for example, during a stomach bug – and can also be used all year round to build up beneficial bacteria; great benefits can be obtained from eating live, natural yoghurt every day. Health food stores also stock probiotic supplements, of which you need to take one or two capsules a day with food. *Lactobacillus acidophilus* and *Lactobacillus bifidus* are good strains for adults.

Hot lemon

Mixed with a little honey and hot water, lemons help soothe sore throats, while also giving you some added vitamin C to help your immune system. Juice four lemons and gently heat in a pan of water, before adding one and a half tablespoons of honey.

Honey

Honey is a popular home remedy in many cultures for coughs and colds. You can take it plain, one teaspoonful at a time, or mix it with some hot water and lemon. A new study in the *Archives of Pediatrics and Adolescent Medicine* provides the first evidence showing that honey may help to calm children's coughs and help them sleep better. Researchers gave 105 children with colds either honey,

honey-flavoured cough medicine or no treatment at all. The children all got better, but honey consistently scored best in parents' rating of their children's cough symptoms. The researchers argue that honey may work by coating and soothing an irritated throat with a substance that has antioxidant and antibacterial effects. Dark-coloured honey, such as the buckwheat honey used in the study, is particularly high in antioxidants. Honey isn't recommended for infants younger than one year old, because of the risk of botulism.

Ginger

Ginger root is another folk remedy for coughs, colds and sore throats. It's used in traditional Chinese medicine to treat coughs, and is also used for colds that are accompanied by a runny nose with a clear nasal discharge, headaches, neck and shoulder aches, and a white tongue coating. In Ayurvedic medicine, the traditional medicine of India, ginger is also used for coughs and colds.

Hot ginger tea is a popular home remedy for cold symptoms and sore throats. Honey and lemon are sometimes added.

Don't fly unless necessary

If you have a cold, there's no point adding strain to your already stressed-out upper respiratory system, which is exactly what the changes in air pressure will do when you fly. Flying with cold or flu congestion can temporarily damage your eardrums as a result of pressure changes during take-off and landing. If you must fly, use a decongestant and carry a nasal spray with you to use just before take-off and landing. Chewing gum and swallowing frequently can also help relieve pressure.

Note: As a rule, make sure you see your doctor if an infection has not responded to natural therapies and has persisted for more than a week. In such cases, antibiotics may be necessary but they should only be used as a last resort (for example, should the illness lead to more serious conditions if left unchecked). Remember that serious conditions such as sinus infections, bronchitis, meningitis, strep throat and asthma can masquerade as a cold. If you have severe symptoms, or feel sicker with each passing day, call your doctor immediately.

Take good care of yourself

Prevention is always so much better than cure. So incorporate as much of the immune-boosting advice given in this book into your life as possible.

If you do find yourself feeling below par, however, or have recently been in contact with someone who has a nasty cold, instead of simply waiting to see if you get ill, take greater care of yourself. If you slow down and pamper yourself a bit, the chances are that your immune system will keep you healthy. And should you catch the odd cold or bug, the symptoms won't drag you down or last nearly as long as they could.

If you think carefully about it, boosting your immunity is really just another way of saying, 'take good care of yourself'. Therefore, be as good to yourself as possible – not just when you feel run down – but all the time. Eating nutritiously, avoiding the enemies of immunity and keeping an active, happy lifestyle will go a long way to giving you the miracle of a robust immune system and the priceless gift of lifelong health.

INDEX